# ASSESSING THE ORAL LANGUAGE DEVELOPMENT AND INTERVENTION NEEDS OF STUDENTS

**Patricia I. Myers**

WITH A CONTRIBUTION BY
Donald D. Hammill

pro-ed
5341 Industrial Oaks Boulevard
Austin, Texas 78735

**The PRO-ED Assessment Series**



*Series Editor*
DONALD D. HAMMILL



**Library of Congress Cataloging-in-Publication Data**

Myers, Patricia I., 1929–
Assessing the oral language development and intervention needs of students.

(The PRO-ED assessment series)
Bibliography: p.
Includes index.
1. Children—Language—Testing. 2. Verbal ability in children—Testing. 3. Handicapped children—Language—Testing. 4. Language disorders in children—Diagnosis. 5. Language acquisition. I. Hammill, Donald D., 1934– . II. Title. III. Series.
LB1139.L3M9 1986 372.6 86-16942
ISBN 0-89079-135-X

pro-ed
5341 Industrial Oaks Boulevard
Austin, Texas 78735

10 9 8 7 6 5 4 3 2 1 87 88 89 90 91 92

# CONTENTS

# PREFACE

The reader can discover many sources dealing with the assessment of oral language, but many of the resources rely on the observation of children in natural settings and on lengthy language or speech samples. In the present book a number of structured techniques for eliciting specific linguistic features are presented. The value of language samples is not denigrated; procuring samples may be the most accurate method of language assessment. However, one must remember that recording and analyzing a language sample is a time-consuming and tedious process for which the public school speech pathologist seldom has the time.

The rationale presented in the book assumes that the speech pathologist has a working knowledge of language development and language structure. The author's belief is that nothing can substitute for such knowledge. Without it, tests or assessment procedures can be of little value beyond their screening capabilities.

The first chapter of the book is an overview of general assessment by series editor Donald D. Hammill. Chapter 2 covers an introduction to the topic of language assessment. Because of the importance assigned to speech and language structure and development, the next two chapters are devoted to these topics. Only a brief review is given, but the reader is referred to a number of more comprehensive references. The last chapter, the lengthiest, is devoted to techniques of informal speech and language assessment.

# 1 / ASSESSING STUDENTS IN THE SCHOOLS

## by Donald D. Hammill

Assessment is the act of acquiring and analyzing information about students for some stated purpose, usually for diagnosing specific problems and for planning instructional programs. This information includes knowledge about an individual's personal attributes, cognitive abilities, environmental status, academic achievement, health, or social competence and is acquired by a variety of techniques of which testing, observation, interviews, record reviews, and analytic teaching are the most frequently used.

The contents of this chapter provide readers with a basic background about assessment concepts and procedures that are currently employed in schools and clinics. Specifically discussed are (a) the purposes for assessing students, (b) the domains of human behavior that are usually measured, (c) the techniques that are most often used to obtain useful information, (d) the frames of reference used to interpret assessment findings, and (e) the role of standardization in assessment.

## PURPOSES FOR ASSESSING STUDENTS

There are important reasons for assessing students. Chief among these are (a) to screen students to find those who need special assistance, (b) to diagnose their problems, (c) to identify their instructional needs, (d) to document their progress in special programs, and (e) to provide information for use in research projects.

## Screening

The first step in a comprehensive assessment program is to locate youngsters who may need special attention. This entails surveying all students enrolled in a school to screen out those who are at risk. Since large numbers of students have to be surveyed, the screening procedures must be time efficient and cost effective.

Generally, two procedures are employed. First, some schools routinely refer for special attention all students who score below a particular level on the group administered readiness or achievement tests that are regularly given. Second, students selected by their teachers as experiencing significant problems may be referred for further study. Children who are identified as somehow deficient through these screening procedures are usually targeted for more in-depth assessment.

## Diagnosing

Diagnosis, originally a medical term, is the recognition of diseases from their symptoms. The physician knows that a fever may be a symptom of many different diseases and that it is necessary to diagnose the disease that is the culprit so appropriate treatment can be prescribed.

In psychoeducational parlance, diagnosis is the use of observed behaviors and events (symptoms) to infer underlying causes and conditions (diagnosis). For example, a child whose speech is characterized by severe word finding problems and unusual syntax, who was late in developing oral language, who has a history of breech birth, and who had a near normal IQ when measured by nonverbal tests (the symptoms) might be labeled as suffering from *specific language disorder* or, as it is sometimes called, *developmental dysphasia* (the diagnosis).

Ideally, a diagnosis should involve not only a label, but also a theory that explains the symptoms. In other words, a diagnosis is the examiner's best estimate of *why* a child acts as he or she does, not a listing or inventory of *what* the child does. For example, to note that Bill is reading four years behind where he should be, given his IQ, is an observation of a symptom, not a diagnosis. To analyze Bill's strengths and weaknesses in reading (e.g., to note that he makes frequent miscues in oral reading, tends to miss inferential comprehension questions, reads slowly, and fails *bl* blends) is nothing more than an elaborate listing of symptoms and should not be considered a diagnosis. Such compendiums of symptoms are useful and contribute to making a diagnosis, but they are not in themselves the diagnosis, because they do not explain why the problems are being evidenced.

Diagnoses may involve organic as well as functional causes. An assessment of Bill, a poor reader, may reveal (a) that reading is not highly prized in his home, (b) that he has many unexcused absences from school, and (c) that he has little interest in learning to read. This particular cluster of symptoms rules out dyslexia (a severe reading problem due to brain dysfunction) as a diagnosis and points to functional causes of Bill's reading problem.

The diagnosis occurs only after the student's academic and behavioral patterns have been determined, the medical, school, and developmental histories have been reviewed, and the parents and teachers have been interviewed. Because of the scope and depth of information that must be interpreted, diagnoses are usually made by multidisciplinary teams. Depending on the nature and severity of the student's symptoms, the team could be composed of any combination of the following: teachers (regular, special, or remedial), physicians, parents, psychologists, speech pathologists, audiologists, optometrists, and physical/occupational therapists, among others.

A diagnosis may or may not be greatly relevant to classroom instruction and planning. To diagnose the problem based on school absences would be highly useful instructionally; however, to classify Sally as autistic tells us little about how to treat her and even less about specific skills she needs to learn. It does, however, influence what might be said to her parents regarding prognosis and expectations and which program she might be referred to for services.

The diagnosis also qualifies Sally for protection under federal and state laws. According to these laws, children diagnosed as having particular handicaps (as in the preceding example, autism) must be served. Undiagnosed children exhibiting similar problems don't have to be served in the schools, even though they may be antisocial, noncompliant, disruptive, abusive, and nonproductive. Under these laws, a clear distinction is drawn between students who are *diagnosed* as having physical, intellectual, emotional, or learning handicaps and those who are not, regardless of their behavior.

## Identifying Instructional Needs

As important as screening and diagnosis are, from the teacher/therapist's point of view, the most useful assessments are those that yield educationally relevant information about a problem. This type of assessment will answer such questions as: Which areas are problematic and which are relatively intact? Which specific skills or behaviors within a problem area are defective or missing? In what order should the defective or missing skills be taught?

**Determining Strengths and Weaknesses.** A comprehensive assessment will determine a student's relative competence in a variety of important areas, especially in the achievement, aptitude, and affective areas. Comparisons of abilities within an area may also be of interest (e.g., within the achievement area, one might assess a student's reading, writing, math, and science proficiency). Even within a single achievement area, such as reading, skill and knowledge comparisons may be made. For example, an examiner occasionally will need to know a student's relative competence among reading comprehension, word recognition skill, phonic and alphabet knowledge, and oral reading rate.

**Selecting Instructional Targets.** While information about a student's general strengths and weaknesses is important, even more detailed information is required before a final comprehensive instructional plan can be generated. For example, the examiner can easily determine the broad content areas in which a student is experiencing problems (e.g., that a child has a problem in math but not in reading). Also, it is a simple matter to recognize that the weakness is centered in subtraction and not in multiplication, addition, or division.

Assuming that a student has difficulty with subtraction, the examiner would need to determine the specific subtraction errors being made. For example, errors might involve problems with borrowing, mistakes due to zero in the minuend, reversals, adding instead of subtracting, ignoring a digit, and so forth. In this case, an analysis of subtraction errors would likely yield content targets that were appropriate for instructional intervention. The correction of these targeted errors becomes an important goal of remediation.

Inherent in selecting instructional targets is attempting to understand the cognitive strategies that the student uses to do school work. Such knowledge has considerable educational and diagnostic importance, because it helps explain why the student makes an error, thereby suggesting how the error can be remediated. For example, Ms. Burton, a third grade teacher, knows from scores on a math test that Jenny ranks in the 10th percentile of mathematical performance, a value indicating a pronounced problem. She knows from direct teaching experience that Jenny fails subtraction problems that require borrowing but passes other kinds of subtraction problems. Now Ms. Burton wants to determine why Jenny has trouble when doing subtraction with borrowing with a problem like $52 - 14 = 42$. Through the use of techniques described in another volume of the PRO-ED Assessment Series, Ms. Burton learns that Jenny's mistake results from her overzealous use of the rule, "Always subtract the smaller from the larger." Thus, Jenny solves the problem by using the following unproductive strategy: She subtracts 2 from 4, since "you always have to take away the small number from the big one." Similar approaches can be undertaken in reading, writing, spelling, speech, and behavior to discover the strategies employed by students to answer questions and solve problems.

**Determining the Sequence of Instructional Tasks.** Having isolated general areas of difficulty and identified specific errors of concern, the examiner must now decide the order in which the errors are to be corrected. In this endeavor, the examiner will find the use of a scope and sequence chart most helpful. On a scope and sequence chart, the broad theoretical categories (the scope) are depicted on one axis, and the skills that comprise the categories (the sequence) are listed in order of development or difficulty on the other axis. A scope and sequence chart displaying the rules governing capitalization and the order (in terms of grade levels) in which they are usually taught is presented in Table 1.1.

**TABLE 1.1. Scope and Sequence of Capitalization**

| | Grade | | | | | | | | |
|---|---|---|---|---|---|---|---|---|---|
| **Words to Capitalize** | **K** | **1** | **2** | **3** | **4** | **5** | **6** | **7** | **8** |
| First word of a sentence | • | • | + | ' | ' | ' | ' | ' | ' |
| First and last names of a person | • | + | ' | ' | ' | ' | ' | ' | ' |
| Name of street or road | • | • | + | ' | ' | ' | ' | ' | ' |
| The word *I* | • | + | ' | ' | ' | ' | ' | ' | ' |
| Name of city or town | | • | + | ' | ' | ' | ' | ' | ' |
| Name of a school or special place | • | • | + | ' | ' | ' | ' | ' | ' |
| Names of months and days | • | • | + | ' | ' | ' | ' | ' | ' |
| First and important words in titles | • | • | • | + | ' | ' | ' | ' | ' |
| Abbreviations: Mr., Mrs., St., Ave. | • | • | + | ' | ' | ' | ' | ' | ' |
| Each line of a poem | | | • | + | ' | ' | ' | ' | ' |
| First word of salutation of a letter | | • | + | ' | ' | ' | ' | ' | ' |
| First word of complimentary close | | • | + | ' | ' | ' | ' | ' | ' |
| Initials | | • | • | + | ' | ' | ' | ' | ' |
| Titles used with names of persons | | | • | • | + | ' | ' | ' | ' |
| First word in an outline topic | | | | • | • | + | ' | ' | ' |
| Names of organizations | | | • | • | + | ' | ' | ' | ' |
| Sacred names | | | • | • | • | + | ' | ' | ' |
| Proper names generally: countries, oceans | | | • | • | • | + | ' | ' | ' |
| Proper adjectives | | | | | • | • | + | ' | ' |
| Titles of respect and rank and their abbreviations | | | • | • | + | ' | ' | ' | ' |

• Introduction; + Suggested teaching; ' Maintenance

From *Experiences in Language: Tools and Techniques* (p. 195) by W. T. Petty, D. C. Petty, and M. F. Becking, 1973, Boston: Allyn & Bacon. Reprinted by permission of the publisher.

If a systematically designed, commercially available program is to be used for instruction (e.g., Silver Burdett's Spelling or SRA's Distar), the examiner should consult the charts that usually accompany such packages. These scope and sequence charts will show both the gross subject matter content areas that are addressed by the program and the specific skills under each for which lessons are provided. Also, entry tests often accompany these programs. Their use will show where the student is performing in terms of the levels and content of the program and, therefore, where to enter the program for the purpose of beginning instruction.

Scope and sequence charts are also available for depicting developmental abilities and skills as well as for subject matter content. These charts are particularly common in the areas of language and motor abilities. Lee (1974) provides an example for spoken grammar. An abbreviated version of her chart is presented in Table 1.2. This particular scope is composed of broad categories of word types, including Personal Pronouns, Main Verbs, Secondary Verbs, Negatives, and so forth. The sequence of skills is grouped into seven developmental levels. The sequence for the Personal Pronouns category begins with first and second personal pronouns (I, you), progresses to third person pronouns (he, she), and continues systematically to plurals (we, us), reflexives (myself, themselves), and *wh-* pronouns (who, which), among others. In scope and sequence charts of this type, the sequence is based on observation of the actual development of children rather than on a purely logical organization of subject matter content.

Often these scope and sequence charts serve as guides in determining the sequence in which needed skills will be taught. For example, from reading a series of essays written by a student, the teacher may identify a set of consistent errors in capitalization. The material in Table 1.1 provides a rationale for listing these errors in preferred order of instruction.

## Monitoring Student Progress

Another important purpose of assessment is to monitor the success or failure of students receiving special attention. It is through such assessments that examiners, teachers, and parents learn whether or not the prescribed intervention has been beneficial. If the student has shown little or no growth or improvement in targeted areas, a change of instructional activities and/or a reevaluation might be appropriate.

Often the documentation of student improvement (or lack of it) is required by law or by school policy. Also, many nonschool agencies make their funding of programs and research contingent upon the testing of students who receive service or who serve as subjects. Even when periodic reassessment is not required, it is a desirable practice to do so, because reassessment provides evidence about whether the instructional program is appropriately meeting the student's needs.

# TABLE 1.2. An Abbreviated Scope and Sequence of Language Training

| Score "Developmental Level" | Indefinite Pronouns or Noun Modifiers | Personal Pronouns | Main Verbs | Secondary Verbs |
|---|---|---|---|---|
| 1 | it, this, that | 1st and 2nd person: I, me, my, mine, you, your(s) | A. Uninflected verb: I *see* you.<br>B. Copula: is or 's: *It's red.*<br>C. is + verb + ing: He *is coming.* | |
| 2 | | 3rd person: he, him, his, she, her, hers | A. -s and -ed: *plays, played*<br>B. Irregular past: *ate, saw*<br>C. Copula: *am, are, was, were*<br>D. Auxiliary: *am, are, was, were* | Five early-developing infinitives<br>I wanna *see* (want to *see*)<br>I'm gonna *see* (going to *see*)<br>I gotta *see* (got to *see*)<br>Lemme [to] *see* (let me [to] *see*)<br>Let's [to] play (let us [us to] *play*) |
| 3 | A. no, some, more, all, lot(s), one(s), two (etc.), other(s), another<br>B. something, somebody, someone | A. Plurals: we, us, our(s), they, them, their<br>B. these, those | | Non-complementing infinitives<br>I stopped to *play.*<br>I'm afraid *to look.*<br>It's hard *to do* that. |
| 4 | nothing, nobody, none, no one | | A. can, will, may + verb: *may go*<br>B. Obligatory do + verb: *don't go*<br>C. Emphatic do + verb: I *do see* | Participle, present or past:<br>I see a boy *running.*<br>I found the toy *broken.* |
| 5 | | Reflectives: myself, yourself, himself, herself, itself, themselves | | A. Early infinitival complements with differing subjects in kernels:<br>I want you to *come.*<br>Let him [to] *see.*<br>B. Later infinitival complements:<br>I had *to go.* I told him *to go.*<br>I tried *to go.* He ought *to go.*<br>C. Obligatory deletions:<br>Make it [to] *go.*<br>I'd better [to] *go.*<br>D. Infinitive with wh word:<br>I know what *to get.*<br>I know how *to do* it. |
| 6 | | A. Wh- pronouns: who, which, whose, whom, what, that, how many, how much<br>I know *who* came.<br>That's *what* I said.<br>B. Wh- word + infinitive:<br>I know *what* to do.<br>I know *who(m)* to take. | A. could, would, should, might + verb *might come, could be*<br>B. Obligatory does, did + verb<br>C. Emphasis does, did + verb | |
| 7 | A. any, anything, anybody, anyone<br>B. every, everything, everybody, everyone<br>C. both, few, many, each, several, most, least, much, next, first, last, second (etc.) | (his) own, one, onself, whichever, whoever, whatever<br>Take *whatever* you like | A. Passive with *get,* any tense. Passive with *be,* any tense<br>B. must, shall + verb *must come*<br>C. have + verb + en *I've eaten.*<br>D. have got *I've got* it. | Passive infinitival complement:<br>With *get:* I have *to get dressed.*<br>I don't want to *get hurt.*<br>With *be:* I want *to be pulled.*<br>It's going *to be locked.* |

From *Interactive Language Development* (pp. 4–5) by Laura Lee, R. A. Koenigsknecht, and S. T. Mulhern, 1975, Evanston, IL: Northwestern University Press. Reprinted by permission.

### Conducting Research

Another purpose of collecting data on students is to participate in research projects. Each year the school district will initiate or cooperate in a number of research projects which will require the testing of students. The results of this research are important to education, especially when they lead to definitive conclusions about the effectiveness of intervention programs, the validity of theoretical positions, the relationship among instructionally relevant abilities, the statistical adequacy of assessment devices and procedures, and the availability of local norms for tests used in the district.

## FREQUENTLY ASSESSED DOMAINS

After an extensive survey of the assessment literature, Hammill, Brown, and Bryant (in press) concluded that almost all of the variables evaluated in schools could easily be grouped under three headings or domains: aptitude, achievement, and affect.

### Aptitude Domain

The term *aptitude* refers to natural capacity, potential, or ability. Most aspects of what is considered general intelligence and the specific mental abilities that are used to measure the concept can fairly be considered aptitudes. Aptitudes are considered to be developmental abilities that are acquired through common, everyday experience. As such, they are present to some degree in all people, unless the individual has physical limitations (e.g., blindness, deafness, cerebral palsy). For example, all people possess some proficiency in language, thinking, or manual dexterity, though they vary widely in their relative competence in these abilities.

In schools, aptitude is generally assessed to obtain an estimate of a student's potential for successful school work. The underlying assumption in aptitude evaluation is that a youngster who has not profited from incidental experience will likely have problems in school mastering formally taught subject matter. Of course, a competent aptitude evaluation will go well beyond merely documenting that a student has not profited from everyday experience by seeking to explain why the student has not profited from such experience.

### Achievement Domain

The term *achievement* refers to those skills that a person has mastered as a result of direct instruction. The skills may be teacher-taught, parent-taught, or self-taught; but they exist only in those individuals who have had specific training. As such, achievement skills (e.g., reading, writing, computer use, alphabet knowledge, or typewriting) are not present in all persons. In the school, achievement assessments are conducted mostly to discover how much a student knows about a particular content, which subskills need to be taught, and what success was attained as a result of instruction.

### Affect Domain

The term *affect* refers to the feelings that people have toward themselves or toward other people, institutions, or ideas. Assessments of this domain in school aged students is done most frequently to secure information about attitudes, interests, and feelings involving school, community, home, peers, work, and self.

Obviously, a comprehensive assessment of a student who evidences a serious problem should include all three domains (aptitude, achievement, and affect). Information pertinent to these domains must be integrated if a student's difficulty is to be diagnosed accurately and if an individual plan of instruction is to be prepared.

## ASSESSMENT TECHNIQUES

In this section, the techniques most frequently used to assess students are described. Any of these techniques can be used to assess any of the domains described above and to achieve any of the purposes previously stated. In the discussions that follow, the emphasis is placed on the use of the techniques for instructional purposes, that is, for obtaining educationally useful information. Six techniques are described: testing, product analysis, direct observation, interviews, analytic teaching, and record review.

### Testing

A test "may be thought of as a set of tasks or questions intended to elicit particular types of behaviors when presented under standardized conditions and to yield scores that have psychometric properties" (American Psychological Association, 1974, p. 2). According to this definition, a wide variety of school assessment techniques would have to be considered tests.

The tasks or questions on a test (usually called *items*) can measure different aspects of a student's academic knowledge, skill mastery, behavior, athletic performance, values, interests, or some other physical, mental, or behavioral attributes. The particular format of these items may vary considerably. On some occasions, a student's knowledge may be tested directly, as on an IQ test or a teacher's daily math test. In these cases, actual competence is measured by having the student answer objective questions, solve problems, and so on.

At other times, checklists and rating scales are used. Items on these tests are statements that are actually inferred questions. These statements or questions are prepared to solicit specific information about a person's opinion or observation of something. Sometimes the user of these tests is a person who is describing the behavior of another person; sometimes a person is describing his or her own behavior. The main difference between rating scales and checklists is that on the rating scale the informant can indicate the degree to which a characteristic is present (e.g., Johnny is absent: rarely, seldom, occasionally, often), while on the checklist the informant is limited to a simple yes or no (e.g., Johnny can count from 1 to 10: yes, no).

The instructions for taking tests may be written or oral; and the responses may require writing, speaking, or performing some action. In responding to items, students may be expected to choose between dichotomous answers (yes-no; true-false), to select an answer from among multiple choices, to give a correct answer to a factual question (Who discovered America?), to compose an essay, to relate a story, to point to answers, or to employ any of countless other possibilities.

Regardless of the test's content or format, its results can be interpreted from a norm, criterion, or nonreferenced point of view. Also, depending on the intention of its author, a test can vary markedly in its degree of standardization. The roles of referencing and standardization are important measurement concepts that determine greatly how assessment results are interpreted. Since these topics are germane to all assessment techniques, they will be discussed in detail later in this chapter.

Readers interested in the procedures, statistical and otherwise, used to construct tests are referred to the comprehensive texts of Anastasi (1982), Gronlund (1985), and Nunnally (1978). For narrative overviews of an exhaustive number of tests, Mitchell's (1985) *The Ninth Mental Measurements Yearbook* is the prime source. When objective critiques of tests' standardization and norming properties are required, Hammill, Brown, and Bryant's (in press) *A Consumer's Guide to Tests in Print* is recommended.

## Product Analysis

A particularly useful assessment technique involves the analysis of samples of students' products. These products may be samples of speech, written material, or math assignments. The strength of this approach is that it allows the examiner to see firsthand the products of a student's performance in spontaneous, everyday situations.

**Speech and Language Samples.** When collecting a speech and language sample, it is often helpful to tape-record the child's vocalizations so they can be analyzed at leisure at another time. It is also wise to collect several samples over a period of a week or so. The samples should deal with different topics and different speech situations. For example, samples of the child describing the contents of a picture, engaged in free social conversation, or responding to direct questions might be obtained.

These samples can be subject to loose or highly structured analyses. For example, examiners may listen to the speech of the child and note the presence or absence of various parts of speech, sentence types, vocabulary items, and grammatical forms using a gross checklist as a guide; or they may use an elaborate, systematic analysis such as the *Developmental Sentence Analysis* offered by Lee (1971, 1974).

**Reading Samples.** A popular method for assessing reading involves the assessment of errors (or "miscues") made by students during oral reading. Students are asked to read aloud printed passages that vary in difficulty. Their oral production is assessed in terms of their approximation of the printed message. All deviations from the printed version are noted and analyzed for significance.

Wiederholt (1985) provides an example in his report on Dori (Figure 1.1). In reading Story 11 from the *Formal Reading Inventory*, Dori mispronounced *indolence* and *procrastination*, substituted /inherited/ for *inherent*, and omitted *tenacious*. She missed three comprehension questions (noted by the check marks immediately below the story). Each departure from print is listed and classified. Other sophisticated systems for analyzing oral reading miscues are provided in Goodman and Burke's *Reading Miscue Inventory* (1972) and Wiederholt and Bryant's *Gray Oral Reading Tests–Revised* (1986).

**Writing Samples.** The analysis of students' spontaneously written material, including stories, letters, and essays, is highly productive from an assessment point of view. These compositions can be assessed from many different perspectives. A glance is all that is necessary to make judgments about legibility and length; more care is needed in conducting a thorough assessment of such factors as proficiency in vocabulary, grammar, syntax, spelling, punctuation, capitalization, and idea expression.

A teacher-diagnostician could have a class or two write a story on some given topic of interest. After reading 30 or so essays on the same topic, the teacher should be quite sensitive to the themes, vocabulary, grammar, and so on, used by most of the students. Departures from modal responses are likely to be of clinical interest. Compositions that make use of dialogue, humor, philosophic or moral themes, complex story sequences, paragraphs, and imagination tend to be more mature than those that do not. The quality of the vocabulary used can be estimated by consulting graded word lists

## FIGURE 1.1. Example of an Analysis of Oral Reading

Student's Name Dori

Form ________ Oral Reading Level 11

### TEACHER'S COPY OF STORY

**Story 11**

Although indolence and procrastination were inherent in Jane's constitution, she prospered in learning through the sheer vigor of her intellect. From an early age she was uncommonly inquisitive, and her memory was so tenacious that her mentors were forever incredulous at her powers of retention. Endowed with boundless and restless mental faculties, Jane read prodigiously but in a desultory manner, and seemed to acquire knowledge by an intuition unbuttressed by the steady application of diligence. In that particular parish, genius had an aura of the divine, and it was axiomatic that anyone with a love of letters was naturally disposed to pedagogy. So when Jane's father found himself in straitened circumstances and Jane was compelled to earn her keep, she was soon engaged as a governess. The truth is, however, that she lacked the patient and methodical nature that would fit her to conduct her charges in learning by gradations. This made it difficult to descend to particulars and mince her precepts for her pupils to swallow.

1. ✓ 2. ____ 3. ✓ 4. ✓ 5. ____

**FIGURE 1.1.** continued

## DEPARTURE FROM PRINT ANALYSIS

Student's Name Dori

Form ________ Oral Reading Level 11

| NO. | LINE | TEXT WORD | MISCUE | Meaning Similarity | Function Similarity | Graphic/Phonemic Similarity | Multiple Sources | Self-Correction |
|---|---|---|---|---|---|---|---|---|
| 1 | 1 | indolence | indolence | 0 | 0 | 1 | 0 | 0 |
| 2 | 1 | procrastination | prostication | 0 | 0 | 1 | 0 | 0 |
| 3 | 1 | inherent | inherited/R | 1 | 1 | 1 | 1 | 1 |
| 4 | 2 | vigor | vigor | 0 | 0 | 1 | 0 | 0 |
| 5 | 4 | mentors | meators | 0 | 0 | 1 | 0 | 0 |
| 6 | 4 | incredulous | incrucials | 0 | 0 | 1 | 0 | 0 |
| 7 | 4 | at | as | 0 | 1 | 1 | 1 | 0 |
| 8 | 4 | retention | reaction/R | 0 | 1 | 1 | 1 | 1 |
| 9 | 5 | boundless | flauntless | 0 | 0 | 1 | 0 | 0 |
| 10 | 5 | prodigiously | porsosly | 0 | 0 | 1 | 0 | 0 |
| 11 | 5 | desultory | desulong | 0 | 0 | 1 | 0 | 0 |
| 12 | 7 | diligence | diligence | 0 | 0 | 1 | 0 | 0 |
| 13 | 7 | genius | genus/R | 0 | 0 | 1 | 0 | 1 |
| 14 | 8 | axiomatic | tomatic | 0 | 0 | 1 | 0 | 0 |
| 15 | 9 | pedagogy | pamady | 0 | 0 | 1 | 0 | 0 |
| 16 | 9 | straitened | stranded | 0 | 1 | 1 | 1 | 0 |
| 17 | 11 | patient | patience | 0 | 1 | 1 | 1 | 0 |
| 18 | 12 | methodical | methoginal | 0 | 0 | 1 | 0 | 0 |
| 19 | 12 | gradations | graderate | 0 | 0 | 1 | 0 | 0 |
| 20 | 13 | descend | resend | 0 | 1 | 1 | 1 | 0 |
| 21 | 13 | to | the | 0 | 1 | 1 | 1 | 0 |
| 22 | 13 | precepts | appropriations | 0 | 1 | 1 | 1 | 0 |
| 23 | | | | | | | | |
| 24 | | | | | | | | |
| 25 | | | | | | | | |
| | | | TOTAL YES | 1 | 8 | 22 | 8 | 3 |
| | | | TOTAL NO | 21 | 14 | 0 | 14 | 19 |

**OTHER MISCUES**

**Type**

- Omissions O ☐
- Additions ∧ ☐
- Dialect ∨ ☐
- Reversals ~ ☐

**OTHER OBSERVATIONS**

**Type**

- Slow reading rate ☐
- Word-by-word reading ☐
- Poor phrasing ☐
- Lack of expression ☐
- Pitch too high or low; voice too soft or strained ☐
- Poor enunciation ☐

**Type**

- Disregard of punctuation ☐
- Head movement ☐
- Finger pointing ☐
- Loss of place ☐
- Nervousness ☐
- Poor attitude ☐
- Other ________ ☐

or by simply noting the number of large words (those with seven or more letters) used in relation to the total number of words in the composition. Analyzing the grammatic character of individual "thought units" or sentences is often used as an estimate of syntactic complexity. Errors in spelling, grammar, punctuation, and capitalization are easy to identify and can be noted for later instruction.

**Math Samples.** The most popular way to assess computation skills involves error analysis using samples of math problems as the basis. It has been noted that students do not tend to make random mistakes. Instead, their errors seem to follow fairly consistent patterns. To this point, Howell and Kaplan (1980) state:

> . . . little information is obtained by simply reporting the number of errors a student makes. The knowledge that "Jenny got five wrong" is not particularly valuable. However, hearing that "Jenny made five multiplication errors and they all involve ×8" could lead you to think that you should teach Jenny her 8's. (p. 245)

In addition to studying the pattern of errors, the teacher may be interested in learning how the student came to make the error. To determine how a student reaches a wrong answer is often a simple task—just ask the student to verbalize the process he or she uses while working out a problem. For example:

| *Problem A* | *Problem B* |
|---|---|
| $\begin{array}{r} 17 \\ +\ 5 \\ \hline 112 \end{array}$ | $\begin{array}{r} 17 \\ +\ 5 \\ \hline 85 \end{array}$ |

While working Problem A, Sally verbalizes, "Seven and five are twelve. Put twelve below the line and bring down the one up there next to the seven. That makes 112." In this problem, she is using a process to solve the problem that she thinks is correct, a process that she likely applies to all similar problems.

While working Problem B, Bill verbalizes, "Seven times five is 35. Put the five below the line and hold the three. Five times one is five. Add three to it and put the eight below the line in front of the five. The answer is 85." He has obviously misread the sign and has multiplied instead of adding.

The error analysis and verbalizing technique is applicable to assessing arithmetic reasoning and geometry skills as well. For readers who wish to know more about error analysis, there are several fine sources, including Ashlock (1976), and Howell and Kaplan (1980). Readers who are interested in a particularly thorough and systematic technique for analyzing math errors are referred to the *Diagnostic Test of Arithmetic Strategies* (Ginsburg & Mathews, 1984).

## Direct Observation

Valuable assessment information about a student can also result from direct observation. In using this technique, targeted students are watched carefully, and their behaviors are noted and analyzed. The data collector (i.e., the observer) can be the classroom teacher or a specially trained person.

Direct observation provides some unique data about a student and is particularly useful when assessing behavior problems, breaches of discipline, acting out behavior, or social maladjustment. Direct observation of the youngster in the classroom can confirm or raise questions about the validity of the referral. Of all the assessment techniques available, this one permits the evaluation of individuals while they are in a natural environment (i.e., when they are functioning in an everyday setting). The technique is also useful in assessing the nature of teacher-student interactions and the classroom climate.

In discussing the reasons for and advantages of direct observation, Wiederholt, Hammill, and Brown (1983) list several:

> First, observation can confirm or disconfirm statements or hypotheses made about the student. Second, patterns of student participation and interaction with people, with tasks, and with objects (such as trading cards, marbles, or furniture) can be noted and documented. A third purpose for observation is to note consistencies and inconsistencies in patterns of behavior, both over time and from setting to setting. Fourth, factors that appear to influence the student's behavior can be identified. And fifth, any student behaviors of concern may be described more accurately as the observer sees what the student actually does. (p. 24)

The manner in which observations are noted varies widely along a nonstructured to highly structured continuum. At one end, the observer might merely watch the student engaged in everyday play or classroom activity and thereby secure an overall picture of the situation. At the other end of the continuum, each of the student's behaviors might be classified and frequencies of occurrence tallied over a specified period of time. On those occasions where student-teacher interactions are being observed, there exist several elaborate systems for recording and interpreting the nature of the interactions noted (Brophy and Good, 1969; Flanders, 1970; Medley, Schluck, & Ames, 1968).

Regardless of how much care is taken in faithfully recording observed behaviors, examiners often become overly subjective in specifying the cause for or the meaning of the behaviors observed. The degree to which an observer can analyze behaviors accurately depends heavily on the training and experience of the observer.

Bloom and Lahey (1978) illustrate this point by giving the example of how a professional jockey and a casual appreciator of horses might view a particular horse. Without doubt, the jockey is in a position to see more, understand more, suspect more, and speculate with more assurance than someone with less experience.

## Interviews

An interview is "a conversation directed to a definite purpose other than satisfaction in the conversation itself" (Bingham, Moore, & Gustad, 1957, p. 3). Because interviews always have a predetermined purpose (i.e., are undertaken to obtain specific information about something), they play an important role in many comprehensive assessment efforts.

Much useful information about students' needs and problems can be assembled by interviewing parents, teachers, and the students themselves. The results of these interviews can be used to study attitudes, perceptions, and feelings about the causes, nature, and consequences of a particular problem area; settings and situations in which problems occur; and countless other nuances associated with a suspected difficulty.

Most teachers value the information derived from interviews and spend considerable time each year talking with and seeking data from parents, students, and other teachers about specific students. The interview approach provides a convenient way of obtaining perceptions that a person has about a situation or event that is current or historic. For example, interviewing the parents of a student with behavioral problems will yield insights into how the student is perceived and treated at home and what the parents believe is causing or contributing to the problems. These perceptions are usually highly idiosyncratic and subjective and, therefore, should not be taken at face value. Yet they do provide the teacher-diagnostician with clues concerning factors that might be influencing a specific situation.

A good interview is not a haphazard undertaking. On the contrary, the interviewer must decide in advance the particular purposes for the conversation, the questions that are to be asked, the most expedient method for initiating the interview, and other pertinent procedural matters. There is a definite art and science to interviewing. Fortunately, there are several useful how-to books available. Among these are books by Stewart and Cash (1985), Gordon (1970), and McCallon and McCray (1975). Of particular interest is Ginsburg (1987), who shows how the interview technique can be applied to instructional assessment, especially math assessment.

## Analytic Teaching

Many assessment oriented practitioners have devised methods of analyzing a student's behavior while the student is engaged in dynamic, ongoing instructional situations. Information from these analyses is used to form hypotheses about the nature of the problem and to determine the next steps in assessment or instruction. The procedure is also used to observe student progress and to discover the elements that need to be changed where expected progress is not evident.

Analytic teaching is known by many names, including "diagnostic teaching," "prescriptive teaching," "directive teaching," "adaptive teaching," and "clinical teaching." All of the systems represented by these terms involve the breaking down of observed behaviors into their component parts so they can be more fully examined for instructional or diagnostic purposes. This is the very essence of the word *analysis* and the reason we prefer to call these systems "analytic teaching."

Wiederholt, Hammill, and Brown (1983) note that analytic teaching methods share at least four characteristics:

> (1) The practitioner has to observe the student engaged in the behavior of interest; (2) the student's responses must be noted and analyzed within some constant frame of reference; (3) the selection of future steps to be taken depends on the interpretation of the results of the successive response analyses; and (4) the methodologies are flexible enough to be applied to almost all aspects of a student's school performance, including academic, linguistic, emotional, and social areas. Methodologies that share these characteristics are grouped under the heading analytic teaching. (p. 32)

Analytic teaching methodologies are exemplified by the clinical teaching techniques of Johnson and Myklebust (1967) and the directive teaching approach of Stephens (1970). The adaptive testing assessment method of Hausserman (1958) is also a technique that combines behavioral analysis of responses with ongoing instruction.

A simple example of an analytic teaching session is provided by Hammill and Bartel (1986) and involves the attempt of a teacher to learn about a student's knowledge of colors. In this instance, the teacher wishes to discover the extent of John's understanding of concepts related to colors. To accomplish this, the teacher probes for answers to the following questions:

1. Can John match the basic colors (place red chips together, blue chips together, and so forth)? If not, what colors does he have difficulty in matching?
2. If asked to point to the red chip, then to the blue chip, and so forth, can John select the correct chip from among others of different colors?

3. If the teacher points to the red chip, then to the blue chip, and so forth and says "What color is this?" does John answer correctly?

These three questions all relate to the general question of whether or not the child can recognize colors, but they also provide different kinds of information about the level of his knowledge, the particular colors he does not know, and how to begin to teach him. First he learns to discriminate among the colors, then he learns the labels (receptive language), and finally he uses the labels in speech (expressive language). (p. 9)

Analytic teaching is particularly useful (a) in detecting areas of weakness and strength; (b) in verifying, probing, or discarding the conclusions and recommendations derived from other sources; (c) in deducing specific instructional or behavioral needs; and (d) in formulating remedial programs. This is accomplished through an ongoing process of teaching the child and analyzing his or her responses to various instructional tasks.

## Reviewing School and Anecdotal Records

The usefulness of reviewing school records, especially as the practice relates to assessment, is described quite adequately in Chapter 2 of *The Resource Teacher* by Wiederholt, Hammill, and Brown (1983). Rather than attempt to "gild the lily," their comments are simply quoted at this time.

The analysis and review of records made about the student is one of the most important of assessment activities, and it is also one of the most overlooked sources of information. Review of records is relatively unobtrusive, is inexpensive, and is one of the major sources of information for generating assessment questions.

Records are often in disarray and may be poorly organized because no one may have taken or been given the responsibility of records collection and organization. When they are not organized, it is impossible to evaluate the relevance of information gathered. People may continue to collect information superstitiously, believing that it is of value when it is not, or they may understandably complain about collecting information that is never used. People rarely mind collecting information that can be shown to be helpful to a student. Especially where the resources for data or information collection are limited, the resource teacher, usually in conjunction with others in the school, will want to make a careful study of the records system.

The kind of information we can expect from a review and analysis of records is reflected in the following questions:

1. What is the nature of the information provided? The information should be relevant to any presenting problems. It should also be comprehensive enough to describe the problem or the student adequately. Both positive and negative information are important. We will also want to know if information that should

be there is missing. This is especially true of information that is needed to rule out possible causes of problems or certain instructional methods. Instructional records often lack enough detail to permit a real analysis of the instructional history of the student.

2. How current is the information? There is no need to duplicate information that is already available. On the other hand, if people are making decisions on old information, there should be an updating to be sure that the information used is currently valid.

3. How reliable and valid is the information? The data base for any statements made about the student must be known. The data base is then evaluated literally as to its goodness. Some statements, such as "John has a central auditory processing disorder, because he mispronounces words such as *chimney* as *chimley* and *came* as *come*," are clearly in need of further interpretation. In addition, statements based upon a one-time observation, or upon only a single setting may be suspect. Observable fact must be separated from professional fiction.

4. What discrepancies about the student or his or her behavior are apparent from the records? These discrepancies may be between one time and another, between one setting and another, or between an expectation and an actual performance. The sudden onset of social, emotional, or academic problems, as well as gradual declines (as in IQ scores) are signals either of invalid information or a serious adverse change in the student or in his or her environment.

5. What consistent patterns of behaviors, comments about the student, or test scores are noted? Consistencies provide some evidence of reliability in information and evidence for the chronic nature of a problem. On the other hand, we would be concerned about the effectiveness of the instructional program if records showed a consistent pattern of no change during any time of remedial effort.

6. How is the information in the records organized? Although this question is not about the student, it has implications both for the wise use of the resource teacher's time and energy and for public relations with those who will be asked to gather information on behalf of the student. When records are not organized, it becomes impossible to evaluate the relevance of the information recorded, and people continue to collect information that is irrelevant or unused.

In addition to the need for organizing records, the form of the organization is important. While there is an apparent advantage in having a purely chronological account of a student, eventually the information should also be reorganized around presenting problems as well. The problem-oriented record described by Weed (1971) is often used in settings where more than one person works with a student or is to observe the student or where the problem is persistent across time and settings.[1]

[1]From *The Resource Teacher* (pp. 23–24) by J. L. Wiederholt, D. D. Hammill, and V. Brown, 1983, Austin, TX: PRO-ED. Reprinted by permission.

## INTERPRETING ASSESSMENT RESULTS

The results of assessment activity, whether test scores, records of anecdotal events, answers to interview questions, or descriptions of performance, are at best merely observations of behavior. To be of maximal use, these findings must be interpreted (i.e., some system must be applied that gives these sterile observations meaning). In general, interpretative systems are of two types: referenced and nonreferenced.

The two most prevalent forms of referenced interpretation are norm referenced and criterion referenced. Both of these referenced systems interpret behavior in terms of some absolute standard existing outside the student. Norm referenced interpretation assumes some idea of normalcy for rating scores. Criterion referenced interpretation involves precisely stated objectives to indicate skill mastery. In addition to these two approaches, this section covers what we have designated nonreferenced interpretation.

### Norm Referenced Interpretation

According to Gronlund (1985), norm referenced interpretations can be applied to all kinds of assessment data and need not be restricted to test derived scores. When norm referenced interpretations are made, a test score or an observed behavior is compared to some real or hypothetical average representation of persons who share common characteristics with the individual being evaluated (the normative referent group). A test score or a particular behavior might be described as being more or less equal to, above, or below the average of the normative sample. Thus, norm referenced interpretations are made to describe interindividual differences among people (i.e., to see how far a person's behavior is from some perceived or statistically determined average).

**Interpretation of Raw Scores.** When norm referenced interpretations are based on test performance, the total number of correct responses (the raw score) made by students in the normative sample are converted to values that truly reflect their distance from the average score of the group. There is a simple procedure for doing this. At each age interval, the raw scores made by students are plotted on a cumulative frequency distribution chart from which percentiles and standard scores are calculated. Percentiles are particularly useful when describing test results to parents, teachers, and the child tested. For example, to say that Phil reads at the 85th percentile means that he performs better than 85 out of a 100 students his age.

The test data derived from the normative sample can also be used to calculate other normative scores, such as age and grade equivalents. Their use results in such statements as Phyllis does math at the 8.5 grade level or Richard is at the second year level in gross motor development. These values are not as accurate as percentiles and standard scores, and their use sometimes can lead to a distorted picture of a child's true abilities. Most authorities recommend strongly that such scores be avoided in school practice.

**Demographic Characteristics of Norm Sample.** The group whose scores are used to compute test norms may represent the national population, students attending school in a particular district, a single classroom of students, or even a class of handicapped people. In any case, test developers are required to show that their normative sample is representative of the desired population. To illustrate, where the reference group is the country's general population, test developers will show that the demographic characteristics of the normative sample are essentially the same as those for the national population. The characteristics might be sex, age, social class, urban-rural residence, geographic area, educational level of parents, and so forth.

The normative referent does not have to be statistically determined or based on some formally identified normative sample. Rather, norms may be based simply on the experience of a teacher, therapist, or examiner. In such a case, a student's performance is compared with the professional's knowledge of how most people the student's age have in the past performed a given task in a particular situation. For example, most competent third grade teachers with ten years classroom experience need no normative tables to tell them what typical behavior is for third graders. It is against this experiential background that the teacher judges an individual student's performance as good, average, or poor.

**The Norm Referencing Process.** Consider four-year-old Sally, who is suspected of being mentally retarded. Mr. Jones, the examiner, could use information obtained from both tests with formally derived norms and other unnormed assessment procedures to reach a norm referenced decision. For example, he could administer the *Detroit Tests of Learning Aptitude–Primary* (Hammill & Bryant, 1986) and use its tables to secure norm referenced data about Sally's intellectual competence.

Next, Mr. Jones could devote an hour or so to observing Sally at free play, asking her questions about the everyday world, watching her interact with other kids, and interviewing her parents. After all of this, Mr. Jones would compare his observations with his knowledge about how children Sally's age usually perform under the conditions that were observed. Here, he is using his "internal norms," norms that are derived from his training and experience, as the basis for interpreting Sally's performance.

Examples of norm referenced statements are listed below.

1. Bob scored at the 23rd percentile on the Graduate Record Exam.
2. Cynthia was third in her class in reading and received an A.
3. Professor Wylie curved the grades on his last test.
4. Six-year-old Willie's behavior was considered poor by his teacher, because he was acting like a four-year-old.
5. The new student did math at the sixth grade level, even though his grade equivalent for his math score on the *Metropolitan Achievement Test* was 4.4.
6. Sam has a two-year discrepancy between his IQ and achievement test score.
7. For her age, she is a very good girl.
8. William scored 23 points in the game, which was four points above the school average.

## Criterion Referenced Interpretation

As is the case with norm reference, criterion reference refers to a method of interpreting assessment findings, a method applicable to all types of assessment techniques, including standardized tests, interviews, and informal teacher made tests. Unlike norm referencing, however, criterion referencing is undertaken to learn what an individual can do unrelated to the performance of others. In other words, student performance is interpreted in an absolute rather than in a relative sense. Sometimes this method is called content, domain, universe, or mastery referencing.

Generally, the domain to be evaluated is clearly defined in terms of skills, tasks, or test items; and the criterion for successful mastery is specified (e.g., the student either passes or fails an activity; he or she can pass an activity 75% of the time). To use an example from Salvia and Ysseldyke (1985), criterion referenced assessments "provide answers to specific questions such as 'Does Maureen spell the word *dog* correctly?' " (p. 30). For such a question, Maureen's spelling proficiency compared to her peers is irrelevant; spelling the word correctly is evidence of her mastery of the task. While the performance criterion in norm referenced interpretation is the average performance of some specified population, in criterion referenced interpretation, the criterion is a predetermined level of performance on some task or series of tasks.

Obviously, criterion referenced assessment has considerable relevance for instruction and is widely practiced in the classroom. It can be used to inventory a student's instructional needs, to monitor success in a program of study, or to place a youngster into a curriculum. Classroom teachers frequently apply this frame of reference to the results of their own classroom tests. For example, on Monday a teacher may give his or her students 20 new words to learn to spell by Friday. On Friday the students are tested. Instances where students spell 17 words correctly are taken as evidence that they have mastered those words on the test. Misspelled words are singled out for special instruction, and the student is retested later on these words.

Examples of criterion referenced statements are listed below.

1. Mary could spell only 5 of the 20 words.
2. Though otherwise proficient, Billy missed 5 of 10 words containing *bl* blends.
3. James has mispronounced words having r's in them in 7 out of 10 trials.
4. Of all the spelling rules, Nell has the most trouble with "i before e except after c."
5. William scored 23 points in the game and was added to the school's athletic Hall of Fame.
6. Having passed 85% of the questions on Form A of the test, the student undertook to answer the questions on Form B.
7. Since Morris made 8 baskets in 10 trials, he qualified for the team.
8. Tom made a B in algebra class.

## Nonreferenced Interpretation

Like norm and criterion referenced interpretations, nonreferenced interpretations also are concerned with what students do. But in this case, the concern is focused on learning what strategies or systems students use to solve problems and reach answers.

Naturally, answers that students give to problems and to teachers' questions, even when incorrect, are not always reached by guessing. Usually, students use what for them seems to be a logical procedure for reaching their answers. Knowledge of these procedures is useful for the examiner, because if the teacher understands how a student has reached an erroneous conclusion or how a student has reached an acceptable conclusion in an inefficient way, it is often an easy matter to provide the student with a new strategy that works better.

**How Nonreferencing Works.** While the other types of referencing have clear-cut criteria for correctness (right-wrong) or mastery (pass-fail), nonreferenced interpretations have no hard and fast rules governing correctness. Consider the example provided in Figure 1.2. By watching students attack the problem or by asking them how they did it, the examiner can easily learn the strategies that were employed to achieve the task. There are many approaches to solving the problem, some more efficient than others, none entirely worthless. For example, one student may count the number of right angles, another student may begin by counting the smaller triangles and work up systematically to the larger ones, another student may take a pencil and shade each triangle after counting it (as a reminder not to count it twice), another student may start counting in the lower left corner and expand to the rest of the figure, and so forth. All of these strategies work to some extent; perhaps some work better for some students than for others. The example provided is a simple one, purposely chosen to show clearly what is meant by nonreferencing and why there can be no rigid criteria for correctness.

**FIGURE 1.2. Triangle Problem**

Task: How many triangles are embedded in this picture?

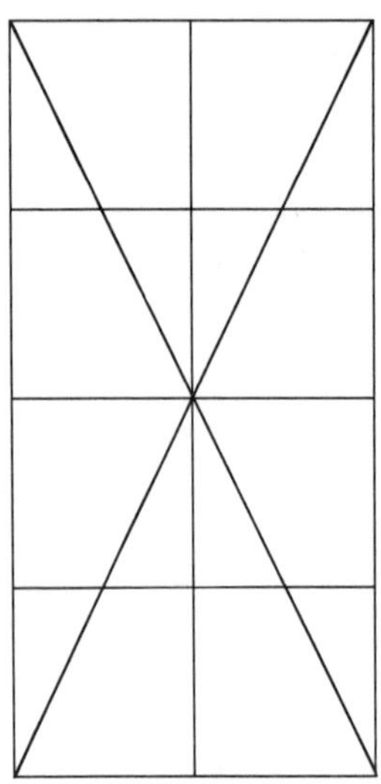

**Nonreferencing as a Designation.** Some authorities might consider nonreferenced interpretation a subtype of criterion referencing. Millman (1974), for example, uses criterion referencing in a very general sense and assigns to that category all absolute interpretations, including even those where no explicit criterion for success is stated and where scores are used for purely descriptive purposes. Most writers, however, do not consider this type of interpretation an example of criterion referencing.

As no name could be found in the literature for this kind of interpretation, I called it *nonreferencing*, recognizing that this term is not completely satisfactory. Perhaps in time a better term will be coined, but for now this one will suffice. Alternative terms were considered (e.g., intrinsic, self, individual, idiosyncratic, strategy, and solution referencing), but all were discarded for one reason or another.

Examples of nonreferenced statements are listed below.

1. David failed to carry in problem 12, and in problem 16 he transposed digits in the remainder.
2. When Lois does something she shouldn't, she always tries to lie her way out of it.
3. William misses many baskets on days when he is criticized by his coach.
4. Mary spells words the way she says them, misspelling the ones she mispronounces.
5. James used the mnemonic device H-O-M-E-S to help recall the names of the Great Lakes.
6. In oral reading, Billy substitutes semantically similar words for words he does not know (e.g., reading aloud "He drove down the road" for "He drove down the thoroughfare").
7. Jan can tell the story better if she has time to rehearse and make notes.

## STANDARDIZED AND NONSTANDARDIZED ASSESSMENT

One frequently reads about the importance of using standardized methods in assessment, but much confusion exists as to what constitutes a standardized method. To help clarify this situation, this section discusses (a) the elements that comprise the concept of standardization, (b) the evidence required to prove that a technique is in fact standardized, and (c) the value of using nonstandardized techniques.

## The Three Elements of Standardized Assessment

Paraphrasing Nunnally (1978) and Anastasi (1982), a well-standardized technique will have clear rules governing its use and will require uniform skills in administering the test and interpreting its results. These are the elements that form the concept of *standardized assessment*. To a considerable degree, it is the presence of these elements that help make reliability and validity of a technique possible. Each element is discussed below.

**Set Administration Procedures.** All standardized assessments include precise instructions governing how the technique is to be administered. These instructions specify a variety of things, including what may be said to the student, what materials are needed, how picture books, blocks, or other physical components are to be managed, when to discontinue the procedure, and many other important aspects required in using a particular technique. Set administration procedures are important to all types of assessments, including tests, interviewing, direct observation, and analytic teaching.

**Objective Scoring Criteria.** Another factor in standardized assessment is the provision of some system for scoring or reporting behavior objectively. If the technique is a test, the system will include specific criteria for what constitutes a correct or incorrect answer. For nontest assessments, other systems are available for noting behaviors, for example, classifying different types of teacher-student interactions in classroom observation situations and recording student comments during or immediately after interviews. In all cases, care is taken to prepare the examiner to see the behavior clearly, to classify it according to some system, and to record it properly.

**A Specified Preferred Frame of Reference.** The authors or proponents of a well-standardized technique will indicate clearly the frame of reference that is best applied to its results. If the technique calls for a norm referenced interpretation, information will be provided for using normative tables or developmental levels. If a criterion referenced interpretation is to be applied, specifications for item mastery will be offered. If a nonreferenced interpretation is the goal, a particular system for classifying errors or identifying strategies will be provided.

In standardized assessment, these guidelines governing administration, scoring, and interpretation are not mere recommendations; they are to be followed to the letter. Adherence to the stated procedures is so important that any divergence is assumed to invalidate the results to some extent. As a consequence of using these guidelines, there is a higher degree of consistency in results among examiners. This is a basic assumption underlying standardized assessment—namely, that different examiners will obtain more or less the same results when using the same procedure. Following the designated procedures minimizes error and increases the probability that what an examiner sees or hears will truly reflect the student's abilities, knowledge, or behavior.

## The Two "Proofs" of Adequate Standardization

Standard administration procedures, standard scoring criteria, and standard means of interpretation represent the very essence of standardization, and it is difficult to see how any assessment technique that did not handle these three elements well could be considered standardized. Yet their presence alone does not ensure that a technique is in fact standardized. To be certain that a technique is properly standardized, the examiner must consider evidence concerning the two proofs of adequate standardization: reliability and validity. Without the availability of convincing evidence regarding these proofs, no technique can be considered adequately standardized.

**Evidence of Reliability.** The experimental demonstration of a procedure's reliability is an important proof of a proper standardization. Unreliable procedures yield untrustworthy results; untrustworthy results lead directly to errors in their interpretation; and errors in the interpretation of results invariably end up producing negative consequences for the individuals who were assessed. There are several sources of error that influence reliability; errors associated with content sampling, time sampling, and interobserver sampling are the most frequently studied.

Content sampling is associated exclusively with the reliability of tests. The amount of error that exists as a function of the items selected to create a test is called content sampling error and is estimated by any of several statistical procedures, including split-halving and application of the Küder-Richardson or coefficient Alpha formulas.

Time sampling is associated with all types of assessment techniques. Error due to the random fluctuations from one assessment session to another is called time sampling error and is usually estimated by the test-retest method.

Interobserver reliability can also be computed on test data but more frequently is used to estimate reliability of other types of techniques (e.g., the analysis of students' written products or speech and language samples). Error due to different observers is called interobserver sampling error and is estimated by intercorrelating the observations or by computing the percentage of agreement among observers.

Most of these methods yield a summative statistic, the reliability coefficient. The magnitude of this coefficient tells how much confidence one should place in the results of a procedure. In the case of interobserver reliability, the percentage of agreement serves this purpose.

**Evidence of Validity.** Simply put, validity refers to the evidence that an assessment procedure measures what it is said or believed to measure. In the case of standardized measurement, the evidence must be thoroughly demonstrated, usually through logical or experimental means. Three kinds of validity are generally considered appropriate for standardized techniques: content, criterion related, and construct.

*Content validity.* Gronlund (1985) writes that "content validation is the process of determining the extent to which a set of test tasks provides a relevant and representative sample of the domain of tasks under consideration" (p. 59). Although Gronlund is writing specifically about tests, his definition can be generalized to all forms of assessment.

Obviously, content validity has to be built into the assessment technique from the beginning. In doing this, great care must be taken to construct test items, interview questions, error analysis systems, and so forth, that adequately represent significant aspects of the domain being assessed.

The content validity of a spelling test could be demonstrated by showing that its items were consistent with the material that is actually being taught in the school. This would be sufficient for a teacher's purposes, but authors of a test built for commercial distribution should go further and demonstrate through item analytic procedures the suitability of their items.

The content validity of a list of questions being prepared for use in an interview to learn a person's interests in a particular occupation could be validated by submitting the list to a panel of practitioners in that field. These practitioners could judge the extent to which the questions reflect significant aspects of their occupation.

The content validity of an error analysis system could be demonstrated by showing that the errors are classified in a way that is consistent with current theory. For example, a system for classifying articulation errors could reflect current ideas about feature analysis, especially relative to place, manner, and voicing. A classification system for oral reading errors might reflect the newer ideas about miscues, especially relative to semantically, phonically, and graphically similar substitutions.

*Criterion related validity.* Criterion related validity is defined as the extent to which performance measured or observed by some procedure is related to some other valued measure of the same performance. This form of validity can be established by using the results to predict future performance or by correlating the results with those from some already accepted procedure. For example, the results of teachers' overall ratings of reading readiness could be used to predict first grade reading success, or the scores from a new test of reading could be correlated with those of an older well-established reading test. Both of these examples provide evidence of criterion related validity.

*Construct validity.* This type of validity refers to the degree to which the underlying constructs of a procedure can be identified and the extent to which these traits reflect the theoretical model on which the procedure is based. Gronlund (1985) offers a three-step procedure for demonstrating construct validity. First, several constructs presumed to account for performance are identified. Second, hypotheses are generated that are based on the identified constructs. Third, the hypotheses are verified by logical or empirical methods. For example, the developers of a new test of reading might as a result of their knowledge of the reading process hypothesize that reading should be related to age (because reading is developmental in nature), to IQ (because reading is a cognitive ability), and to grades (because reading is a key skill helpful in all academic subjects). If the new test did correlate highly with age, IQ, and grades, it would be evidence that the new test possessed construct validity. Though this example pertains to the construct validity of a test, the concept is equally applicable to the results of all kinds of assessment techniques.

**Conclusion.** In concluding this discussion about standardization, three important points should be made. First, even though the majority of the evaluation literature discusses standardization almost exclusively in terms of its relation to tests, the reader should recognize that the elements and proofs represent important generic concepts in measurement. As such, they are applicable to all assessment techniques and should not be restricted to tests. To be sure, knowledge of reliability and validity is as critical to interpreting data acquired from interviewing, observing, and analytic teaching as it is to interpreting data acquired from testing.

Second, the reader will note that the presence of norms is not included among either the elements or the proofs of standardization. While norms are often associated with highly standardized devices, especially those built for the expressed purpose of making norm referenced interpretations, their presence is by no means an essential criterion for standardization. Many assessment techniques are perfected specifically for research uses or for making criterion or nonreferenced interpretations. In such instances, norms are superfluous. Yet these procedures need precise administration instructions, reliable results, and consistent interpretations as much as those intended for norm referenced use.

Third, assessment techniques can easily be classified into three groups—highly standardized, standardized, and nonstandardized—according to their degree of standardization in terms of the previously described proofs. Techniques for which exhaustive evidence (e.g., multiple studies) is available that shows acceptable reliability and validity can fairly be called *highly standardized.* Techniques that have only minimal evidence (e.g., one or two studies showing acceptable reliability and validity) qualify for a *standardized* rating. Techniques for which no proof of reliability or validity is available, only nonsupportive evidence exists, or evidence is provided for only one of the two proofs must be considered *nonstandardized.* In general usage, *formal* is used as a synonym for "standardized" or "highly standardized"; *informal* is used as a synonym for "nonstandardized."

## The Value of Nonstandardized Techniques

The advantages of using well-built, highly standardized techniques are obvious: Their use yields reliable and valid results, the kind of results that are most needed for justifying placement decisions about students and for documenting growth. But a high price often is paid for this standardization; for example, the examiner's freedom to improvise and to probe is sacrificed, the breadth and depth of the content assessed has to be restricted or arbitrarily fixed, and the setting in which the assessment takes place has to be contrived to satisfy the demands expected of standardized techniques.

To prepare instructional plans for students and to diagnose their problems properly, examiners frequently need information that lies outside the purview of standardized assessment. Sometimes examiners want to assess areas for which standardized techniques are simply not available. Sometimes they want to probe the extent of a student's knowledge of a subject in ways that are impossible under standardized conditions. The three examples that follow show how the use of nonstandardized procedures can produce relevant, useful assessment information.

**Example #1.** If the student doesn't understand what is asked of him or her, the examiner can reformulate the instructions to a simpler level and try again. If the student still doesn't understand, the examiner can demonstrate over and over again until the student finally gets the idea.

**Example #2.** Knowledge of whether or not students misspelled this or that word or failed a particular task is not as important for many purposes as trying to learn why they did not achieve as expected and determining the conditions under which they might have performed well. For example, when students give the wrong answer to a problem, the examiner could (a) tell them to be more careful and to do the problem again, (b) call their attention to particularly relevant elements in the problem before asking them to attempt it a second time, or (c) ask them how they came to the answer that was given. Knowing how a student's performance is altered on an assessment task under each of the conditions listed may have significant educational implications.

**Example #3.** On a given day, Ms. Foster, a fifth grade teacher, may decide to test her students' mastery of multiplication, because it has been the subject of instruction for the past week. She prepares a test in which the problems require knowledge of those aspects of multiplication that had been taught. Usually she makes up the problems to be included on the test; occasionally the problems are drawn from workbooks, teacher's manuals, or other classroom sources. It is Ms. Foster's personal judgment about the need for and relevance of the information to be assessed that determines the nature of the items placed on the test. Without doubt, the teacher has used some rationale in constructing her test, but she will rarely see the need or have the desire for expressing it formally.

The flexibility in administering, scoring, and interpreting procedures evidenced by these examples is simply not permitted when using standardized procedures. Yet the examples illustrate how instructionally important assessment information can result from the use of nonstandardized procedures. Surely the findings obtained through nonstandardized techniques are not substitutes for those derived from standardized methods, but they can augment such findings and from the teacher's point of view are often infinitely more valuable.

## CONCLUSION

Finally, there are four questions that examiners should consider carefully when thinking about assessment. These are the Whys?, Whats?, Whiches?, and Hows? that underlie the understanding of all assessment efforts.

1. Why is the assessment being undertaken? Is it done to diagnose students, to document progress, or to acquire instructionally relevant information?
2. What is going to be measured—that is, which attributes in the achievement, aptitude, or affective domains are the targets for assessment?
3. Which of the available assessment techniques are to be employed: tests, interviews, analytic teaching, direct observation, review of records, or analysis of student production?
4. How are the resulting data to be interpreted? Are they going to be subjected to a norm, criterion or nonreferenced interpretation?

## REFERENCES

American Psychological Association. (1974). *Standards for educational and psychological tests.* Washington, DC: Author.

Anastasi, A. (1982). *Psychological testing* (5th ed.). New York: Macmillan.

Ashlock, R. B. (1976). *Error patterns in computation.* New York: McGraw-Hill.

Bingham, W., Moore, B. V., & Gustad, J. W. (1957). *How to interview.* New York: Harper & Row.

Bloom, L., & Lahey, M. (1978). *Language development and language disorders.* New York: John Wiley.

Brophy, J. E., & Good, T. L. (1969). *Teacher-child dyadic interaction: A manual for coding classroom behavior.* Austin, TX: Research and Development Center for Teacher Education. The University of Texas.

Flanders, N. (1970). *Analyzing teaching behavior.* Menlo Park, CA: Addison-Wesley.

Ginsburg, H. P. (1987). *Assessing the arithmetic abilities and instructional needs of students.* Austin, TX: PRO-ED.

Ginsburg, H. P., & Mathews, S. C. (1984). *Diagnostic Test of Arithmetic Strategies.* Austin, TX: PRO-ED.

Goodman, Y., & Burke, C. L. (1972). *Reading Miscue Inventory.* New York: Macmillan.

Gordon, T. (1970). *Parent effectiveness training.* New York: Wyden.

Gronlund, N. E. (1985). *Measurement and evaluation in teaching* (5th ed.). New York: Macmillan.

Hammill, D. D., & Bartel, N. (1986). Meeting the special needs of children. In D. D. Hammill & N. Bartel (Eds.), *Teaching students with learning and behavior problems* (pp. 1–21). Austin, TX: PRO-ED.

Hammill, D. D., Brown, L., & Bryant, B. (in press). *A consumer's guide to tests in print.* Austin, TX: PRO-ED.

Hammill, D. D., & Bryant, B. (1986). *Detroit Tests of Learning Aptitude–Primary.* Austin, TX: PRO-ED.

Hausserman, E. (1958). *Developmental potential of preschool children.* New York: Grune & Stratton.

Howell, K. W., & Kaplan, J. S. (1980). *Diagnosing basic skills.* Columbus, OH: Charles E. Merrill.

Johnson, D., & Myklebust, H. (1967). *Learning disabilities: Educational principles and practices.* New York: Grune & Stratton.

Lee, L. (1971). Developmental sentence scoring. A clinical procedure for estimating syntactic development in children's spontaneous speech. *Journal of Speech and Hearing Disorders, 36,* 315–331.

Lee, L. (1974). *Developmental sentence analysis.* Evanston, IL: Northwestern University Press.

Lee, L., Koenigsknecht, R. A., & Mulhern, S. T. (1975). *Interactive language development.* Evanston, IL: Northwestern University Press.

McCallon, E., & McCray, E. (1975). *Planning and conducting interviews.* Austin, TX: Learning Concepts.

Medley, D., Schluck, C., & Ames, N. (1968). *Assessing the learning environment in the classroom: A manual for users of OSCAR 5.* Princeton, NJ: Educational Testing Services.

Millman, J. (1974). Criterion-referenced measurement. In W. J. Popham (Ed.), *Evaluation in education. Current applications* (pp. 309–397). Berkeley, CA: McCutchan.

Mitchell, J. V. (Ed). (1985). *The ninth mental measurements yearbook.* Lincoln, NE: The University of Nebraska Press.

Nunnally, J. S. (1978). *Psychometric theory* (4th ed.). New York: McGraw-Hill.

Salvia, J., & Ysseldyke, J. E. (1985). *Assessment in special and remedial education* (3rd ed.). Boston: Houghton Mifflin.

Stephens, T. M. (1970). *Directive teaching of children with learning and behavior handicaps.* Columbus, OH: Charles E. Merrill.

Stewart, D. J., & Cash, W. B. (1985). *Interviewing: Principles and practices* (4th ed.). Dubuque, IA: Brown.

Wiederholt, J. L. (1985). *Formal Reading Inventory.* Austin, TX: PRO-ED.

Wiederholt, J. L., & Bryant, B. (1986). *Gray Oral Reading Tests–Revised.* Austin, TX: PRO-ED.

Wiederholt, J. L., Hammill, D. D., & Brown, V. (1983). *The resource teacher.* Austin, TX: PRO-ED.

# 2 / AN OVERVIEW OF LANGUAGE ASSESSMENT

The assessment of children's language abilities and disabilities has been a preoccupation of speech pathologists, psychologists, and other appraisal personnel for well over twenty years. Psycholinguistic models of assessment enjoyed great popularity with such professionals during the 1970s and gave rise to a number of standardized tests—some more related to language than others—such as the *Illinois Test of Psycholinguistic Abilities* (ITPA) (Kirk, McCarthy, & Kirk, 1968), the *Utah Test of Language Development* (Mecham, Jex, & Jones, 1978), and others. During this time, content validity was asserted by simply using face validity as evidence that psycholinguistic abilities were measured by a test. The extensive use of these tests means that the assessment process has become vested in a model that yields little in-depth information regarding a child's language abilities (Muma, 1983).

Already enchanted with psychometric models, professionals in language assessment became equally entranced with Chomsky's theories of generative grammar. If these professionals considered themselves too progressive to continue using the ITPA, they simply exchanged it for some other instrument, such as the *Developmental Sentence Analysis* (Lee, 1974) or one of the developmental profiles. However, the 1970s began with the "semantic revolution" heralded by Bloom (1970), Bowerman (1973a), Schlesinger (1971), and Slobin (1973) and ended with the "pragmatics revolution" led by Bates (1976a), Bates et al. (1979), and Dore (1975). As Leonard (1983) notes, the gains made in the 1970s were solidified by the substantive data that became available at that time and by expanded knowledge about the learning of language.

This knowledge will continue to bring about profound changes in all aspects of language and its assessment. For example, assessment and treatment procedures focusing on psycholinguistic abilities or on grammar must be altered radically to reflect the discovery that the linguistic structure of children's speech is determined by the dual needs to be meaningful and to have some social effect.

Chapter 5 discusses assessment procedures, including the value of traditional measures of articulation, grammar, and other language abilities. There are children with only articulation problems, children who need improved vocabularies, and children in need of syntactic refinements. For those children, the conventional assessment procedures will serve. However, more and more children with severe language disorders are being seen in our schools and clinics—children who are retarded, autistic, or in some other way severely deficient in language—for whom the traditional approaches to assessment and remediation are seriously inadequate.

Any discussion of language assessment must deal with at least four major areas: the assessment framework, the nature and structure of language, the development of language, and the specific assessment procedures. Because this book is devoted to assessment for instructional purposes, the assessment framework is discussed first. The work of Chapman (1976), Miller (1978, 1981), and Muma (1983) has provided a basis for many of the concepts in this book.

The approach to assessment set forth in this book is fundamentally developmental. It focuses on defining and describing the developmental status of the child for each of the basic language processes: comprehension, production, and communication. These processes are discussed in Chapter 3 under the more traditional categories of phonology, syntax, semantics, and pragmatics. Regardless of the taxonomical problems in describing language, the following problems in assessment must be considered.

- It is difficult to quantify many of the elusive aspects of deviant language.
- Developmental data are often incomplete, fragmented, and sometimes inconsistent.
- Theories and models of language behavior are often too narrow, too broad, vary greatly from one another, or simply ignore deviant language.
- Many excellent approaches to assessment are too time-consuming to be employed outside of an experimental situation.

These difficulties must be accepted. One must assume a positive approach to assessment, accept the challenge, and attempt to apply what is known, what is best, and what is feasible.

The most efficient approach to assessment is attempting to answer the three questions posed by Miller (1978):

1. Why are we assessing the child?
2. What are we going to assess?
3. How are we going to assess the child? (p. 273)

The answer to any of the questions will affect the others, because they are interactive, relating to each other in a reciprocal fashion. For example, if assessment is being done because the child has a functional articulation disorder, the "what" and "how" are to some extent predetermined.

## WHY ASSESS LANGUAGE?

Obviously, children's language is assessed to discover whether their language behaviors are deviant and, if so, to what degree. However, assessment involves much more than the designation of "problem/no problem" that arises when someone questions the child's language behavior with regard to its quantity or quality. The basic aim of assessment is deceptively simple; it implies that one will be able to establish the normalcy or deviance of the child's language and that one knows what constitutes normal language behavior in a 3 year old or an 8 year old. In the past, clinicians have relied upon standardized norm referenced tests to provide the answers to these questions. However, severely language delayed or disordered children presently being referred for assessment are unable to respond to the requirements of a standardized testing situation. Moreover, research is indicating more and more that language development can be highly idiosyncratic and that what is normal for most children may not be normal for the individual child.

A second reason for assessing the child's language is to provide baseline information regarding the different components of language. The establishment of baseline functioning enables the evaluator to estimate the developmental level at which children are performing by comparing their performances to test norms or to developmental data. The existence of a developmental delay or disorder can be established only after the child's developmental level is determined. It should be noted here that there is little agreement on the terms *language delay* and *language disorder*. Some authors equate the two terms (Coggins, 1976; Miller & Yoder, 1973; Morehead & Ingram, 1973), but others differentiate them, using the rationale that some children are delayed in language acquisition but are progressing in normal sequence, while other children's development is violating the sequence at least insofar as that sequence is known (Bax & Stephenson, 1977; Cousins, 1979; Menyuk, 1968).

A third reason for assessment, and the most important from the viewpoint of the clinician, is to provide information for the design and development of a therapeutic program. The data gathered in the assessment can determine the developmental level at which therapy should begin and aids the clinician in determining which processes and components of language should be included in the therapy program. Although the treatment of language disorders is not within the purview of this text, it should be noted that the baseline information obtained in assessment is important in determining whether progress is being made by the child and at what rate the progress, if any, is occurring.

## WHAT IS TO BE ASSESSED?

The elements, the components, the processes of language are to be assessed, and determining what those elements are forms the basis of the answer to the question, "What?" The reader will find that language is discussed throughout the text in terms of four components: phonology, syntax, semantics, and pragmatics. As mentioned earlier, it would be possible to categorize the content of assessment into the same elements as those of language or to use other divisions, such as the processes of language: comprehension, production, and pragmatics. It is also possible to use the first categorization system and, with the exception of pragmatics, break down the components into their receptive and productive aspects.

Another aspect of language that must be preserved in assessment is the complexity of language. The field of language assessment is notorious for the use of quick and easy tests of "simple" processes. One of the reasons given for the use of such tests is that large numbers of children must be assessed, and, therefore, easily-administered instruments are necessary. The difficulty arises when these tests are used for diagnostic purposes and when therapeutic programs are designed based on the results. Unfortunately, some professionals who know better use and advocate such tests which violate a fundamental principle of language therapy by reducing language to simple, and sometimes irrelevant, dimensions.

## HOW TO CONDUCT AN ASSESSMENT

The third question to be asked before assessing a child is, "How am I going to go about the assessment?" This may be the most difficult question of the three, because there are more obstacles and pitfalls in selecting instruments and in eliciting appropriate responses than there are in the other two areas of problem identification and language taxonomy. Assessment procedures can be divided into at least four basic categories: standardized tests, developmental scales, nonstandardized tests, and behavioral observations.

## Standardized Tests

Miller (1978) gives a particularly lucid and succinct definition of a standardized test when he says that it

> . . . is one that has been given to large numbers of children from various populations, has demonstrated reliability (internal and/or test retest), is valid as determined by external or face-validity criteria, and has normative data that provide either scale-score, age-equivalent, or numerical-score comparisons for individual children tested. (p. 291)

Some of the commonly used standardized tests of language are: the *Illinois Test of Psycholinguistic Abilities* (Kirk, McCarthy, & Kirk, 1968), the *Test for Auditory Comprehension of Language* (Carrow, 1973), the *Test of Language Development–Primary* (Newcomer & Hammill, 1982) and *Intermediate* (Hammill & Newcomer, 1982), the *Clinical Evaluation of Language Functions* (Semel & Wiig, 1980), the *Test of Adolescent Language* (Hammill, Brown, Larsen, & Wiederholt, 1987), and the *Carrow Elicited Language Inventory* (Carrow, 1974). Standardized tests are discussed further in chapters 1 and 5.

Standardized tests of language have numerous drawbacks with regard to comprehensive assessment for purposes of program planning. They are seldom, if ever, appropriate for children under 3 years of age, and they are not always appropriate to all populations. In selecting a standardized test, one should search for agreement among the procedures of the test, the child's behavior, and the goals of assessment. Availability of a test is never an adequate substitute for suitability; there are many alternatives to standardized tests.

## Developmental Scales

Developmental scales sample the child's major performance areas across a developmental period and are administered to determine the specific developmental level the child has attained. The scales are only as good as the milestones in development they sample, and a prospective user should examine these milestones very carefully. Sometimes the behaviors sampled are not sequenced discretely enough to allow the examiner to determine at what level the child is really functioning. One behavior at age 2.0 years followed by another at age 3.0 gives the examiner a very cloudy picture of what is going on between ages 2 and 3. Examiners using developmental scales should be grounded in knowledge of language development as thoroughly as possible.

Some of the developmental scales used in schools and clinics are: the *Developmental Activities Screening Inventory* (Fewell & Langley, 1984), the *Minnesota Child Development Inventory* (Ireton & Thwing, 1972), the *Birth to Three Developmental Scale* (Bangs & Dodson, 1979), and the *Utah Test of Language Development* (Mecham, Jex, & Jones, 1978). Developmental scales may require the examiner to check off specific tasks the child is asked to perform or may involve indirect reporting by parents.

## Other Assessment Procedures

The last two types of assessment procedures include the use of partially standardized tests and simple behavioral observations. Tests of language having less than complete standardization include language sample analysis, elicited production, comprehension, and elicited imitation (Miller, 1981). The procedures have a comfortable degree of face validity, suggested administrative procedures, and systems for interpretation, but, more important, they allow for flexibility and modification. As Miller (1978) remarks, these partially standardized tests conform to the child rather than requiring the child to conform to them. A number of these procedures will be discussed in greater detail in the section on assessment procedures (Chapter 5).

Behavioral observation is critical to all types of assessments from standardized to the most nonstandardized of testing to the assessment of specific behaviors in controlled or unstructured, naturalistic situations. Observing a child's behavior requires only meticulous listening, observing, and recording of that behavior, and the results are sometimes considered nonevidential and pedestrian. However, if the literature on the language acquisition process is surveyed, one can conclude without doubt that most of the data on language production have been obtained through observation. As Miller (1978) states, we must know the goals of observation more specifically than with any other type of assessment, as there is no goal inherent in the procedure. "We must know what we are looking for in order to observe the occurrence, frequency, antecedent, and consequent events, and contingencies of specific behaviors of interest" (p. 304).

In summary, assessment must be conducted with a developmental approach, the goal being to assess language behavior directly through the components of phonology, syntax, semantics, and pragmatics and through the language processes of acquisition and use. We should be most interested in what the child is able to do rather than what his or her disabilities are, and we should be even less interested in the labels that test results can provide.

## REFERENCES


Bangs, T., & Dodson, D. (1979). *Birth to Three Developmental Scale.* Dallas: Developmental Learning Materials.

Bates, E. (1976a). *Language and context.* New York: Academic Press.

Bates, E. (1976b). Pragmatics and sociolinguistics in child language. In D. Morehead & A. Morehead (Eds.), *Normal and deficient child language* (pp. 411–463). Austin, TX: PRO-ED.

Bates, E., Benigni, L., Bretherton, I., Camaioni, L., & Volterra, V. (1979). *The emergence of symbols: Cognition and communication in infancy.* New York: Academic Press.

Bax, M., & Stephenson, P. (1977). Analysis of a developmental language delay. *Proceedings of the Royal Society of Medicine, 70,* 727–728.

Bloom, L. (1970). *Language development: Form and function in emerging grammars.* Cambridge, MA: MIT Press.

Bowerman, M. (1973a). *Early syntactic development: A cross-linguistic study with special reference to English.* Cambridge, MA: Cambridge University Press.

Bowerman, M. (1973b). Structural relationships in children's utterances: Syntactic or semantic? In I. E. Moore (Ed.), *Cognitive development and the acquisition of language* (pp. 346–378). New York: Academic Press.

Carrow, E. (1973). *Test for Auditory Comprehension of Language.* New York: Teaching Resources.

Carrow, E. (1974). *Carrow Elicited Language Inventory.* New York: Teaching Resources.

Chapman, R. (1976). Eliciting answers to questions: The development of question comprehension in pre-school children. In J. Miller (Ed.), *Procedures for assessing children's language: A developmental process approach* (p. 450). Madison, WI: Waisman Center on Mental Retardation and Human Development, University of Wisconsin.

Coggins, T. (1976). Early semantic development in retarded children. Unpublished doctoral dissertation, University of Wisconsin, Madison, WI.

Cousins, A. (1979). Grammatical morpheme development in an aphasic child: Some problems with the normative model. Paper presented at the 4th Annual Boston University Conference on Language Development, Boston, MA.

Dore, J. (1975). Holophrases, speech acts, and language universals. *Journal of Child Language, 2,* 21–40.

Fewell, R., & Langley, M. (1984). *Developmental Activities Screening Inventory.* Austin, TX: PRO-ED.

Hammill, D. D., Brown, V., Larsen, S., & Wiederholt, J. L. (1987). *Test of Adolescent Language.* Austin, TX: PRO-ED.

Hammill, D. D., & Newcomer, P. (1982). *Test of Language Development–Intermediate.* Austin, TX: PRO-ED.

Ireton,H., & Thwing, E. (1972). *Minnesota Child Development Inventory.* Minneapolis, MN: Behavior Science Systems.

Kirk, S., McCarthy, J., & Kirk, W. (1968). *The Illinois Test of Psycholinguistic Abilities.* Urbana, IL: University of Illinois Press.

Lee, L. (1974). *Developmental Sentence Analysis.* Evanstan, IL: Northwestern University Press.

Leonard, L. (1983). Discussion: Part II: Defining the boundaries of language disorders in children. In J. Miller, D. Yoder, & R. Schiefelbusch (Eds.), *Contemporary issues in language intervention* (ASHA Reports 12, pp. 107–115). Rockville, MD: American Speech-Language-Hearing Association.

Mecham, M., Jex, J., & Jones, J. (1978). *Utah Test of Language Development.* Austin, TX: PRO-ED.

Menyuk, P. (1968). The role of distinctive features in children's acquisition of phonology. *Journal of Speech and Hearing Research, 11,* 138–146.

Miller, J. (1978). Assessing children's language behavior: A developmental process approach. In R. Schiefelbusch (Ed.), *Bases of language intervention* (pp. 269–319). Austin, TX: PRO-ED.

Miller, J. (1981). *Assessing language production in children: Experimental procedures.* Austin, TX: PRO-ED.

Miller, J., & Yoder, D. (1973). Assessing the comprehension of grammatical form in mentally retarded children. Paper presented at the International Association for the Scientific Study of Mental Deficiency, The Hague.

Morehead, D., & Ingram, D. (1973). The development of base syntax in normal and linguistically deficient children. *Journal of Speech and Hearing Research, 16,* 330–352.

Muma, J. (1983). Speech-language pathology: Emerging clinical expertise in language. In T. Gallagher & C. Prutting. (Eds.), *Pragmatic assessment and intervention issues in language* (pp. 195–215). San Diego, CA: College-Hill Press.

Newcomer, P., & Hammill, D. D. (1982). *Test of Language Development–Intermediate.* Austin, TX: PRO-ED.

Schlesinger, I. (1971). Production of utterances and language acquisition. In D. Slobin (Ed.), *The ontogenesis of grammar* (pp. 63–101). New York: Academic Press.

Semel, E., & Wiig, E. (1980). *Clinical evaluation of language functions: Diagnostic battery examiner's manual.* San Antonio, TX: Psychological Corporation.

Slobin, D. (1973). Cognitive prerequisites for the development of grammar. In C. Ferguson & D. Slobin (Eds.), *Studies of child language development.* New York: Rinehart, Holt, and Winston.

# 3 / THE NATURE AND STRUCTURE OF LANGUAGE

The arguments and professional debates are endless regarding which characteristic, capacity, or ability sets humans apart from the other animals. There are proponents of the opposable thumb, advocates for the ability to problem solve, those who would argue for the capacity to think in abstract terms, and many of us who believe that the one uniquely human capacity is the ability to acquire, develop, use, and continuously expand a verbal symbol system. To those who view a linguistic system as the only characteristic possessed by humans alone, the attempts at teaching language to other primates are feeble experiments in what is little more than sign behavior and rank fairly close to the highly trained animal's ability to follow very complicated signals provided by a trainer.

Human infants do not have to be taught to comprehend and use a linguistic system; they have only to be exposed to an environment in which spoken language is used. Unless children are seriously impaired, probably having a severe to profound hearing loss or a severe dysfunction of critical neurological functions, they will speak the language of their families and communities. Children with mild problems may experience some delay or dysfunction in their linguistic abilities—delays that may be cumulative as they become older. However, humans acquire and use a verbal symbol system that is governed by sets of rules that are phonological, syntactic, and semantic. They use the system in a practical fashion, dependent upon the context, and are never formally taught the system rules until they enter school. By that time the child's basic language, at least in its spoken form, has already been learned, and the only ensuing development is in the direction of enhancing and enriching the child's linguistic system.

Mention was made above of phonological, syntactic, and semantic rules of language. As these are not yet household terms, some explanation of the components of the linguistic system and of its development is in order. The following section provides only a summary of the nature, structure, and development of language; however, ample references are given so that the reader who wishes to pursue a particular topic in depth may do so.

Most authorities in linguistics arbitrarily divide language into three major components: phonology, syntax, and semantics. Others elaborate somewhat on this division and speak of morphology as an element of both syntax and semantics. In recent years, a number of authors discuss pragmatics as a linguistic component separate and apart from syntax and semantics. For our purposes, we will deal with the three major components of phonology, syntax, and semantics and will subsume pragmatics under semantics.

## PHONOLOGY

Phonology refers to the three components of the speech-sound system of a language: segmental features, the rules for combining the segmental features, and supra-segmental features. The segmental features of the sound-system are the phonemes—the discrete speech sounds—of the language; the rules for combining phonemes are known as phonological rules; and the supra-segmental features are the intonational or prosodic elements of speech. Menyuk (1972) provides a lucid example of the three components of phonology by comparing two sentences:

$S_1$ She's a white housekeeper.
$S_2$ He's a lighthouse keeper?

On the segmental—or phonemic—level, a native English speaker distinguishes the difference between *sh/e's* and *h/e's* and between *wh/ite* and *l/ight* because of the differences in the phonemes that form the first segments of the words. Jakobson, Fant, and Halle (1963) hypothesize that these differences are perceived because each phoneme is made up of a particular bundle of distinctive features based on articulatory and acoustic characteristics. Theoretically there is a pool of universal features from which all of the speech sounds of all languages are drawn. One feature that is demonstrated in the two example sentences is the consonantal feature that divides consonants from vowels and from the glides (h, y, w). In the example sentences, *white house* can be distinguished from *lighthouse*, because the latter possesses the consonantal feature, whereas the former does not. Some other distinctive features include the quality of voicing, sibilancy, nasality, and so on. It is possible to plot each phoneme on a table of features, thereby distinguishing each from the other.

Menyuk's two sentences probably would be distinguished from each other first on the supra-segmental level; the speaker would immediately recognize that one is a statement, while the other is a question, because they differ in their fundamental frequency contours. The statement sentence has a falling fundamental frequency contour, and the question has a rising contour. The voice drops at the end of a statement; it rises at the end of a question. There is also a difference in stress in the two sentences. In the first sentence, the stress falls on the syllable *house* in *white housekeeper*, whereas the stress in the second sentence is the syllable *light* in *lighthouse*. The difference in the stress patterns indicates that in $S_1$ the speaker is referring to a housekeeper who is white, while in $S_2$ the reference is to a keeper of a lighthouse.

The phonological rules operating in the two sentences are similar with regard to certain sequential rules. For example, in both sentences the vowel in *she's* and *he's* is lengthened, because the final strident consonant is voiced (pronounced with laryngeal tone). The stop consonants /k/ and /p/ are aspirated in both sentences; if they were not, the segment *keeper* would sound like *geeper*. Many phonological rules govern the articulatory and acoustic characteristics of vowel-consonant, consonant-vowel, and consonant-consonant production in the English language. Of course, other languages use different rules, which is why it is difficult for speakers of one language to produce accurately the phonemic strings of another language. Some of the very common rules that most of us recognize once they are called to our attention are:

- Initial cluster consonants can take only the form of consonant + /w/, /r/, or /l/ unless the consonant is /s/.
- Tense, number, and possession indicated by the addition of *s* or *es* take the following phonomic forms:
    - /z/ after voiced phonemes—play + /z/, tree + /z/, bum + /z/
    - /s/ after unvoiced phonemes—muff + /s/, rat + /s/, dip + /s/
    - /Iz/ after stridents—rose + /Iz/, pass + /Iz/, crash + /Iz/
- Tense indicated by the addition of *ed* takes the following forms:
    - /d/ after voiced phonemes—pay + /d/, sign + /d/, glove + /d/
    - /t/ after unvoiced phonemes—kick + /t/, muff + /t/, rough + /t/
    - /Id/ after /t/ and /d/ phonemes—pat + /Id/, side + /Id/

In evaluating articulatory disorders, the following information about the phonological system is critical and must be known by the individual who undertakes such an assessment:

- Phonetic transcription of the 43 or so phonemes
- Phonological features that distinguish phonemes in words
- Rules for combining matrices of features
- Prosodic features of sentences

The information is critical, because articulation disorders generally result from a failure in one or more of the last three areas, and appraisal must be related to those areas if the results are to be of any value in a therapy program. It goes without saying that the therapist must be able to transcribe in written form exactly what the child is producing, and, therefore, a knowledge of phonetic transcription is vital to preserving a record of articulation proficiency.

## SYNTAX

Syntax is the branch of grammar that is concerned with the arrangement of words in sentences and with the means by which such relations are shown (e.g., word order or inflection). An important element of syntax is morphology, which is the study and analysis of the structure of words, particularly the forms and classes of words (e.g., declensional endings like walk*s*, walk*ed*, or walk*ing* and derivational endings like the *ness* in *goodness*. Morphological analysis is used to describe the grammatical elements in a language by observing their form and function, their phonological variants, and their distribution and mutual relationships within larger stretches of speech.

This section covers three main topics: innate capacity for language, competence versus performance, and the linguistic rules of grammar. Much of the information comes from Noam Chomsky, who revolutionized the study of linguistics, the study of child acquisition and development, and the approaches to remediation of childhood language disorders. The linguistic theory based on Chomsky's work is known as transformational-generative grammar and has been expanded by such authors as Lyons (1968), Postal (1968), Burt (1971), Fowler (1971), Fillmore and Langendoen (1971), and King (1969). Chomsky criticized the traditional schools of linguistics as being merely taxonomic; that is, as simply labeling and listing phonetic, grammatical, and other units of language, thereby neglecting the underlying processes of human speech. According to Chomsky, the object of linguistic analysis must be to discover those elements in language that are universal and regular in the human's innate ability to understand and produce new "grammatical" sentences, even though the individual may never have heard those specific sentences before.

## Innate Capacity

The debate regarding the innate quality of human characteristics has been carried on for years, and the "nature-nurture" arguments are too extensive to recapitulate. Let us say that linguistics and psychologists study the process of language learning by comparing input with output, that is, by comparing the language an infant or young child is exposed to with the language he or she in turn produces. Exactly how the brain is structured to acquire language competence is not known, but the term *language acquisition device* (LAD) was applied by Chomsky (1957) to the unknown function shown in the model below.

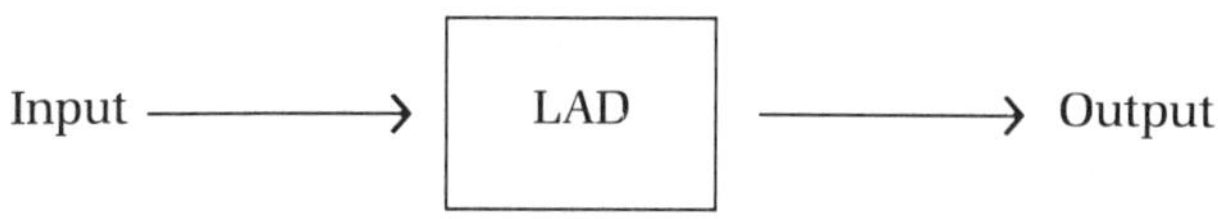


Language is learned and is not instinctive; however, Chomsky and others regard it as an innate capability that requires only the triggering of a speaking environment for its development. More recently, some researchers working in the area of pragmatics have questioned the existence of the LAD and have placed much greater emphasis on the "nurture" aspects of language acquisition.

## Competence Versus Performance

Also implicit in transformational-generative grammar is the concept of competence as opposed to performance. The distinction was drawn originally by Chomsky but has been studied by numerous other linguists and psychologists. Competence refers to the ability that all native speakers have of being able to understand and produce sentences they have never heard before; in this sense, competence refers to the code that underlies all utterances in a given language. On the other hand, performance refers to the utilization of this code in situations where language is used. In transformational-generative grammar, competence features are represented in the deep structure, whereas features of performance are represented in the surface structure. Deep structure is produced by the syntactic component of the grammar, and surface structure is produced by the phonological component. Competence and performance have been likened to a symphony in which competence is the underlying musical rules of tonality, harmony, and so on, and performance is the production that the listener hears.

Grammar in the above sense must account for all the sentences that may be formed in a language and judged correct according to the linguistic intuition of native speakers. At a somewhat deceptively simple level, this intuition can be demonstrated in very young children, who will accept as an English word *splik* but will reject *jrik*. Their linguistic intuition tells them that one is "correct" but that the other is not, even though they have never heard either word nor have they been taught any of the acceptable phonetic combinations of English.

## Linguistic Rules

According to Chomsky, the sentence is the basic unit of language, and he describes relationships between items in the structure of a sentence in terms of abstract statements called *phrase structure rules* and *transformation rules*. A phrase structure rule is a series of syntactic rewrites (can be rewritten as instructions). The rules generate strings and assign a structure to the string. Each rule is in the form of an expansion rule with only one symbol to the left of the arrow; for example, S → NP + VP, which means that a sentence has the structure of a noun phrase (NP) plus a verb phrase (VP). The particle NP → Det + Nom means that a noun phrase consists of a determiner (such as an article) plus a nominal.

$$\text{VP} \longrightarrow \left\{ \begin{array}{l} \text{Vt + NP} \\ \text{Vi} \end{array} \right\}$$

means that the verb phrase consists of transitive verb plus a noun phrase or an intransitive verb standing alone. If these rules are applied, one by one, in the following order:

| | | |
|---|---|---|
| 1. S ⟶ | NP + VP | (A sentence is a noun phrase plus a verb phrase.) |
| 2. NP ⟶ | Det + Nom | (A noun phrase is a determiner plus a nominal.) |
| 3. VP ⟶ | {Vt + NP / Vi} | (A verb phrase is a transitive verb plus a noun phrase or an intransitive verb alone.) |

a series of strings such as the following could be produced:

1. NP + VP (The boy + kicks the ball.)

2. NP + Vt + VP (The boy + kicks + the ball.)

3. Det + Nom + Vt + (The + boy + kicks + the + ball.)

From the examples given above, the reader can see the words form a lexicon (dictionary), and the application of appropriate morphophonological rules produce the sentence, "The boy kicks the ball." The generation of such a sentence can be represented diagrammatically as

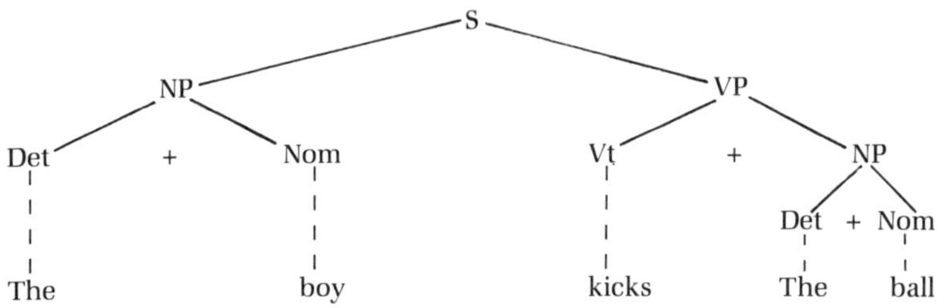


When all of the phrase structure rules have been applied, the result is a terminal string.

In addition to phrase structure rules, Chomsky postulated transformational rules which lay down procedures for converting one grammatical pattern into another. Such a rule may change one sentence type into another, delete or add elements, change the order of elements, or substitute one element for another. Transformational rules operate on the output, that is, the terminal string of the phrase structure rules. As one example, observe the transformation of a declarative sentence into an interrogative sentence. The rule applied is: NP + Pas + be + X ⇄ Pas + be + NP + X, in which Pas = past tense, NP = noun phrase, and X = any construction. Application of the rule results in the following:

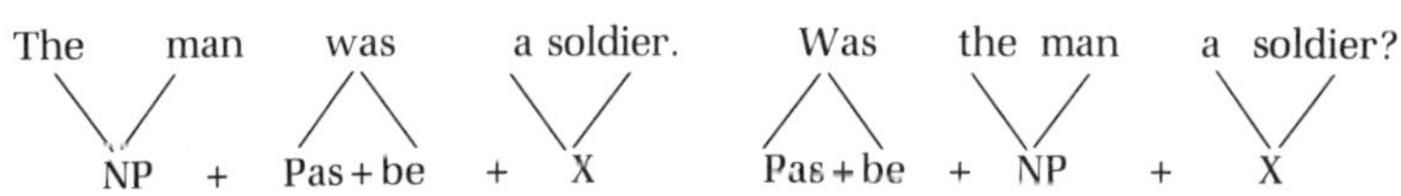


The reader can see that the phrase structure rules describe the basic structures of the language concerned, whereas more complicated structures lend themselves to description as transformations of basic structures by means of transformation rules. In the earliest type of transformational-generative grammar, the rules themselves are usually referred to in terms of three components: first, the *phrase structure component*, consisting of phrase structure rules; second, the *transformation component*, producing strings of formatives (bound morphemes such as prefixes, suffixes, etc.); and third, the *morphophonemic component*, which is a series of rules converting the string of formatives into a phonetic representation.

Before discussing the semantic component of language, a few additional words should be said about morphemes, because a great deal of research has dealt with the acquisition and development of morphological elements. A *morpheme* is a minimum distinctive unit of grammar and, in fact, has been called the smallest unit of meaningful language. A word is composed of one or more morphemes. Like phonemes, a morpheme is a formal element, and a particular morpheme may be represented by different variants (or *allomorphs*) in different environments. For example, the English plural morpheme often symbolized as $s_2$ may occur as /-s/ in cats, /-z/ in dogs, or /iz/ in horses. Because the morpheme is the smallest unit of meaningfulness, a word like *home* cannot be divided into its constituent parts such as *h, ho, ome, me,* and so forth, without the original meaning being lost or changed. Thus, *home* represents a single free morpheme—free, because it can stand alone. The plural morpheme /-s/, along with others, is said to be a bound morpheme, because it can occur only in conjunction with another morpheme.

## SEMANTICS

In Chomsky's later publications (1968), he added a semantic component to the transformational-generative grammar, because he had come to the conclusion that meaning should have the same formal treatment as grammar. Semantics was then included as an integral part of the grammatical analysis of language. The emphasis in transformational-generative grammar is on the elaboration of a logically consistent theory that can explain adequately and formulate explicitly the deep structures of sentences.

In the discussion of semantics, four major areas are discussed: the relationship between the semantic and grammatic components, the referential features of semantics, the semantic features, and the relational features. The first section deals primarily with the work of Chomsky and other transformational grammarians, while the latter sections draw from the work of other theorists.

### Semantics and Grammar

The grammatical relationships inherent in the elements of a phrase or sentence but not immediately apparent from their linear sequences are referred to as the deep structure or, infrequently, the deep grammar. Consider the following English sentences:

1. John expected mother to bring a present.
2. John persuaded mother to bring a present.

The surface structure of the two sentences is identical, as they both consist of Nominal + verb + nominal + marked infinitive + determiner + nominal, but the deep structure of the two sentences is quite different, as can be seen by the fact that the first can be transformed as follows:

3. John expected that mother would bring a present.

However, the second cannot be similarly transformed:

4. John persuaded that mother would bring a present.

Diagrammatically, the difference between the two sentences can be shown as follows:

1. John expected mother to bring a present.

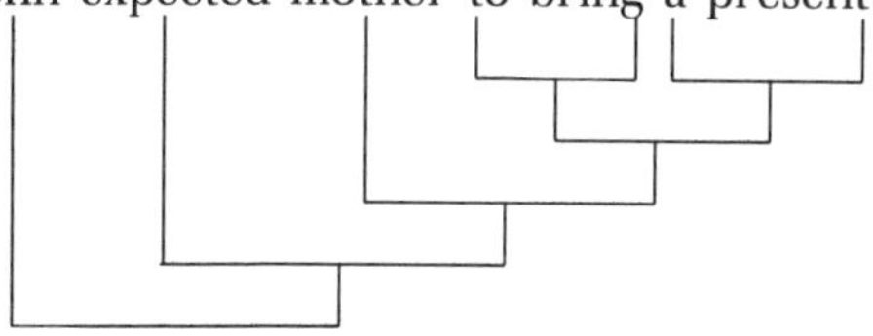

2. John persuaded mother to bring a present.

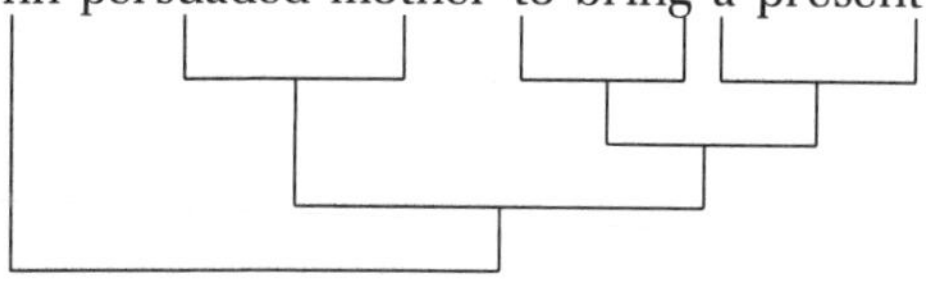

From the above diagrams it can be seen that the difference lies in the nature of the relationship of the verbs *expected* and *persuaded* with the words that follow them. In sentence 1, *expected* is directly related to all of what follows; in sentence 2, *persuaded* is related only to *mother*. In summary, we may say that transformational grammarians view semantics as a study in logical relationships.

Many authors have found the transformational-generative semantics difficult to apply when dealing with acquisition, development, and disorders of language, and the theories have never enjoyed the popularity and discipleship that the theories related to phonology and syntax have had. Leaving the work of Chomsky and other strict transformational linguists, one may define the semantic system of a language as the knowledge that a native speaker must have to understand sentences and to relate them to his or her knowledge of the world. Such a definition obviously implies a strong cognitive element, and many writers in the area of semantics acknowledge their debt to Piaget, Bruner, and other cognitive psychologists.

Semantics includes the knowledge of lexical items individually as well as the meaning of a sentence as determined by the meanings of both the individual lexical items and the structure of the sentence. Lexical items are simply units of the vocabulary of a language—such as words, phrases, or terms—as listed in the dictionary. They usually have a pronounceable or graphic form, fulfill a grammatical rule in a sentence, and carry semantic meaning. It is increasingly apparent that semantics deals with meaningfulness and that a fourth component of language—namely, pragmatics—is more or less embedded in it. For purposes of clarity, pragmatics is discussed in the following section as a component apart from semantics, but, as with all of the language components, that is a highly artificial division.

## Referential Features

One of the earliest theories of semantic meaning is the referential theory in which the meaning of a word is simply its referent or that object to which the word points. In this theory, words are symbols that stand for something other than themselves; for example, *table* refers to a particular piece of furniture, *cat* to a particular animal, *blue* to a particular range of colors, and so on. This is all simple and attractive. However, we also have to account for the meanings of words like *at, but, is,* and other words that have no immediate referents, as well as words that have more than one referent (e.g., *you*) and those that have referents that are difficult to identify (e.g., *unicorn*). Proponents of the referential theory have attempted to deal with words like those above, but as Alston (1964) notes, the explanations raise even more problems.

If every object in the world had exactly one name and every name had only a single referent, it would be much simpler to explain the meaning of meaning. The problem, as pointed out by Brown (1973), is that almost all names actually refer to categories, and every object can be named by a variety of terms. For example, the word *cat* refers to all four-legged animals of a certain type, and the terms *furry creature, tabby,* and so on, all refer to cats. Learning about the referents of words is actually a matter of learning about how human beings organize the world about them.

## Semantic Features

Katz and Postal (1963) and Katz (1966) propose the best known theory for understanding semantic development. (See Chapter 4 for a detailed discussion of language development.) Katz and Postal hypothesize that the meaning of a word consists of two parts: its semantic features and its selection restrictions. Semantic features, of which each word may have several, express parts of the meaning of the word. For example, *cat* has the following features, in addition to many others: *living, animal, four-legged, furry, purring,* and so on. The word *dog* has the same set of features as those given for *cat*, with the exception of *purring*, for which *barking* could be substituted. Dale (1976) lists some of the semantic features of the words *bachelor* and *wife* and illustrates how the term *bachelor's wife* violates the selection restrictions, because *bachelor* includes the feature *unmarried*, while *wife* includes the feature *married*.

### Relational Features

Norman, Rumelhart, and their research group (1975) take issue with the notion that the meaning of a term is the sum of its semantic features. They believe that relational information is also necessary. In considering the word *pay*, one must take into account not only the semantic features of the word but also the relations among the *payer*, the *payee, money, giving,* and *obligation*.

There are numerous other theories and subtheories regarding the nature of semantics, but the majority of the work that has been done in the area focuses on the semantic functions of words within the context of an utterance. For example, Slobin (1970) classifies early two-word utterances in terms of whether they express need, possession, location, and so on, and he finds striking similarities in the types of utterances used by English, Finnish, Russian, German, Luo, and Samoan children. Brown (1973) concentrates on the acquisition of morphology, while performing detailed semantic analyses, and comes to the conclusion that new morphological markers are acquired only after the child knows their underlying semantic distinctions.

## PRAGMATICS

Until the 1970s, much of the research in linguistics, language acquisition, assessment, and therapy focused on grammar and syntax. In the 1970s and early 1980s, authors tended to highlight two facts about language performance—that language always occurs in a context and that contexts are not all the same. Regrettably, these two facts frequently have been seen as obvious and possibly trivial. As Cook-Gumperz and Gumperz (1978) point out, the issue is not that contexts exist or that they vary, but whether contexts are static backgrounds within which language occurs, "a 'label' for a cluster of extralinguistic or extra-grammatical factors" (p. 5), or whether they are dynamic aspects for both the speaker and the listener. Pragmatic theories of language address language as it is used and characterize both linguistic and contextual elements as parts of one interactive communicative whole (Austin, 1962, Bates, 1976a; Searle, 1969). Hymes (1971) speaks of competence for use or communicative competence and points out that equating competence with the speaker/hearer's knowledge of the grammatical rules of language is a narrow view that neglects a body of observable data that depends on rules for the appropriate use of utterances in relevant contexts. Hymes further states that to give a full account of the facts we need an explanation of what the speaker/hearer knows about who can say what, in what way, where and when, by what means, and to whom.

## Theories of Language Pragmatics

The pragmatics of language is vitally concerned with who can say what, as indicated by Hymes. However, earlier researchers such as Morris (1938) discuss the relationship between signs and their interpreters. More recently, Lakoff (1972) states that it is essential to take extralinguistic contextual factors in account, and Bates (1976b) defines pragmatics of language as rules governing the use of language in context. Halliday (1975) relates the structure of language to its individual and social functioning. Searle (1969) discusses the four basic components of how understanding between communicative beings is accomplished:

- the utterance act—uttering words
- the propositional act—referring and predicating
- the illocutionary act—stating, questioning, asserting, etc.
- the perlocutionary act—the effects such acts have on the beliefs, thoughts, actions of the hearer

Searle's classification has been used by Prutting and Kirchner (1983) in developing a pool of pragmatic behaviors for assessment purposes.

Duchan (1983) states that pragmatic knowledge leads to the choice of linguistic structures but does not affect their packaging. According to Bates and MacWhinney (1983), who call their approach *functionalism*, pragmatics is the deepest level of activity in language performance. Because they feel pragmatics provides a foundation for choosing linguistic forms, it seems that pragmatics would be the first aspect or component of language for them to consider. It would precede phonology, syntax, and semantics and, probably, underlie all other components. Duchan (1983) agrees that the change of focus from viewing language form as more significant than the intent behind the form contains the impetus for moving away from a structuralistic, multilevel view of language to a more dynamic, functionalistic model. According to Duchan's theory, the barriers between the components of language (phonology and syntax, syntax and semantics, etc.) would be disregarded in favor of emphasizing the structures within each component. These structures could be classed together in terms of the functions they serve.

## Decoding Speech

Let us return for a moment to Searle's (1969, 1975a, 1975b) description of the *speech act*, a term closely associated with his work. He states that the same sentences may be used as different speech acts. For example, the sentence, "It's almost lunchtime," can serve as a statement of fact; however, if it is said in hope that the listener will provide lunch, it functions as a request. Rees (1978) uses the example of Grandmother's sentence made while sitting with her family at the dining table, "Has everyone had enough?" How do her listeners know that she is saying that she would like someone to pass the food so she can have a second helping? It is certainly not a message that is conveyed by a syntactic/semantic analysis of the utterance. How, in fact, does any listener manage to comprehend any speaker's intentions when the message is conveyed indirectly? Searle (1975a) suggests:

> In indirect speech acts the speaker communicates to the hearer more than he actually says by way of relying on their mutually shared background information, both linguistic and nonlinguistic, together with the general powers of rationality and inference on the part of the hearer. (pp. 60–61)

If a listener is to decode the intended meaning of a sentence, a listener must be able to decide on a particular set of circumstances or prior information to which the information in the heard sentence is related (Rees, 1978). Sometimes the related information is in a previous sentence. Transcriptions of dyadic conversations reveal quite readily that sentences often make no sense unless the reader relates them to the context and to previous sentences in the sample. Freedle and Carroll (1972) give a cogent and lucid example of the interpretation of relations:

> Suppose Frank and Joe are walking down the street and are about to pass a hamburger stand. Frank says, "Would you like to eat here?" Such a question contains assumptions of at least time and space: The time is not "right now" but "pretty soon, after we get served," and the place is not "right here on the street" but "at the counter of the hamburger stand." Yet if Frank and Joe are walking in the park and carrying a picnic basket, the question "Would you like to eat here?" we would assume that the time is "right now, as soon as we unload the basket" and the place could be "right here." In either case, the total situation supplies the context which evokes the semantic assumptions that are most consistent with the utterance. (p. 361)

In addition to context and previous sentences providing interpretive clues to the meaning of a sentence, so do cultural expectations and pragmatic presuppositions (Bates, 1976b). For example, the sentence, "Can you zip me up, honey?" carries with it some very definite cultural expectations for most of us. We would expect that the speaker is a woman and that the listener is a man, a close woman friend, or possibly a child. Rarely would we expect that the listener and speaker are both men. If we hear the sentence, "Could you turn the TV down?" we would be likely to come to one of two conclusions: (a) The speaker and listener are social equals or (b) the speaker is socially superior to the listener but was reared to be polite to social inferiors. However, decide for yourself what the pragmatic presuppositions are for the form of the same sentence, "Turn the TV down!"

### The Cooperative Principle

Another facet of pragmatics, which Grice (1975) calls the cooperative principle, deals with the principles or rules of conversation. He identifies four maxims, or rules, and subrules that listeners and speakers expect each other to observe. These are extracted and simplified by Rees (1978):

A. Quantity (the quantity of information to be provided)
   1. Make your contribution as informative as is required (for the current purposes of the exchange).
   2. Do not make your contribution more informative than is required, or your listener will be misled or think you talk too much.

B. Quality (try to make your contribution one that is true)
   1. Do not say what you believe to be false.
   2. Do not say that for which you lack adequate evidence.

C. Relation (be relevant, whatever that may turn out to mean, specifically)

D. Manner (be perspicuous)
   1. Avoid obscurity of expression.
   2. Avoid ambiguity.
   3. Be brief (avoid unnecessary prolixity).
   4. Be orderly. (p. 207)

## SUMMARY

Language is a highly complex, species-specific, continually developing characteristic of the human being. In this chapter language has been discussed in its phonological, syntactic, semantic, and pragmatic aspects. However, the reader should remember that these divisions of language are artificial and that each aspect of language has a significant and dramatic impact on the others. Although the development of language is discussed in the next chapter using the same divisions as those given above, no pretense is made that the different components are separate or that each can be assessed or treated apart from the others.

## REFERENCES

Alston, W. (1964). *Philosophy of language.* Englewood Cliffs, NJ: Prentice-Hall.

Austin, J. (1962). *How to do things with words.* Cambridge, MA: Harvard University Press.

Bates, E. (1976a). *Language and context.* New York: Academic Press.

Bates, E. (1976b). Pragmatics and sociolinguistics in child language. In D. Morehead & A. Morehead (Eds.), *Normal and deficient child language* (pp. 411–463). Austin, TX: PRO-ED.

Bates, E., & MacWhinney, B. (1983). Functionalist approaches to grammar. In L. Gleitman & E. Wanner (Eds.), *Language acquisition: The state of the art* (pp. 126–154). New York: Cambridge University Press.

Brown R. (1973). *A first language: The early stages.* Cambridge, MA: Harvard University Press.

Burt, M. (1971). *From deep to surface structure: An introduction to transformational syntax.* New York: Harper and Row.

Chomsky, C. (1968). *The acquisition of syntax in children from 5 to 10.* Cambridge, MA: MIT Press.

Chomsky, N. (1957). *Syntactic structures.* The Hague: Mouton.

Cook-Gumperz, J., & Gumperz, J. (1978). Context in children's speech. In N. Waterson & C. Snow (Eds.), *The development of communication* (pp. 214–238). New York: John Wiley.

Dale, P. (1976). *Language development: Structure and function* (2nd ed.). New York: Holt, Rinehart and Winston.

Duchan, J. (1983). Language processing and geodesic domes. In T. Gallagher & C. Prutting (Eds.), *Pragmatic assessment and intervention issues* (pp. 83–101). San Diego: College-Hill Press.

Fillmore, C., & Langendoen, D. (Eds.). (1971). *Studies in linguistic semantics.* New York: Irvington.

Fowler, R. (1971). *An introduction to transformational syntax.* London: Routledge.

Freedle, R., & Carroll, J. (1972). Language comprehension and the acquisition of knowledge: Reflections. In R. Freedle & J. Carroll (Eds.), *Language acquisition and the acquisition of knowledge* (pp. 361–368). New York: John Wiley.

Grice, H. (1975). Logic and conversation. In P. Cole & J. Morgan (Eds.), *Syntax and semantics, Vol. 3: Speech acts* (pp. 43–59). New York: Academic Press.

Halliday, M. (1975). *Learning how to mean: Explorations in the development of language.* London: Edward Arnold.

Hymes, D. (1971). Competence and performance in linguistic theory. In R. Huxley & E. Ingram (Eds.), *Language acquisition: Models and methods* (pp. 3–24). New York: Academic Press.

Jakobson, R., Fant, G., & Halle, M. (1963). *Preliminaries to speech analysis.* Cambridge, MA: MIT Press.

Katz, J. (1966). *The philosophy of language.* New York: Harper and Row.

Katz, J., & Postal, P. (1963). *An integrated theory of linguistic descriptions.* Cambridge, MA: MIT Press.

King, R. (1969). *Historical linguistics and generative grammar.* Englewood Cliffs, NJ: Prentice-Hall.

Lakoff, R. (1972). Language in context. *Language, 48,* 907–927.

Lyons, J. (1968). *Introduction to theoretical linguistics.* London: Cambridge University Press.

Menyuk, P. (1968). The role of distinctive features in children's acquisition of phonology. *Journal of Speech and Hearing Research, 11,* 138–146.

Menyuk, P. (1972). *The development of speech.* New York: Bobbs-Merrill.

Miller, J. (1981). *Assessing language production in children: Experimental procedures.* Austin, TX: PRO-ED.

Morris, C. (1938). *Foundations of the theory of signs.* Chicago: University of Chicago Press.

Norman, D., Rumelhart, D., & the LNR Research Group. (1975). *Explorations in cognition.* San Francisco: Freeman.

Postal, P. (1968). *Aspects of phonological theory.* New York: Harper and Row.

Prutting, C., & Kirchner, D. (1983). Applied pragmatics. In T. Gallagher & C. Prutting (Eds.), *Pragmatic assessment and intervention issues in language* (pp. 29–65). San Diego: College-Hill Press.

Rees, N. (1978). Pragmatics of language: Applications to normal and disordered language development. In R. Schiefelbusch (Ed.), *Bases of language intervention* (pp. 191–269). Austin, TX: PRO-ED.

Searle, J. (1969). *Speech acts.* London: Cambridge University Press.

Searle, J. (1975a). Indirect speech acts. In J. Morgan & P. Cole (Eds.), *Studies in syntax and semantics. Vol. 3: Speech acts* (pp. 133–169). New York: Academic Press.

Searle, J. (1975b). Speech acts and recent linguistics. In D. Aaronson & R. Rieber (Eds.), *Developmental linguistics and communication disorders* (pp. 45–61). New York: Academy of Sciences.

Slobin, D. (1970). Universals of grammatical development in children. In G. Flores d'Arcais & W. Levelt (Eds.), *Advances in psycholinguistics* (pp. 48–61). Amsterdam: North Holland Publishing.

# 4 / THE DEVELOPMENT OF LANGUAGE

In assessing spoken language proficiency, it is desirable that the examiner understand both the structure and the acquisition of language. When nonstandardized testing is done, it is especially important that examiners have a working knowledge of the development of language. They cannot rely on normative data as is provided by standardized tests but must depend on information about the sequential development of spoken language and the approximate ages at which various structures emerge. Many of the strategies discussed in Chapter 5 are only vaguely age-referenced, but they are presented in sequence.

When do children acquire and develop adult oral language? In the early and mid 1960s, researchers concentrated on the development of the formal structures of language. In the 1970s, they moved on to investigate the semantic structures underlying the morphophonemic and syntactic structures. By the late 1970s to the present, the greatest interest has been in how language is acquired. In addition, the study of pragmatic aspects of language acquisition has greatly increased in recent years. In this chapter, acquisition and development in their phonological, syntactic, semantic, and pragmatic aspects are discussed, although it should be emphasized again that it is actually impossible to divide language into separate, discrete components. All components are interrelated, and the reader will see later in this chapter when Brown's research on development is discussed that there is definite overlap between syntactic and semantic development.

## PHONOLOGICAL DEVELOPMENT

The first reviews of speech sound acquisition and development dealt with the ages at which various phonemes were acquired by young children. Tables of development were generated by numerous authors, and general agreement was found among those authors (Davis, 1938; Irwin, 1947, 1948; Templin, 1957). The results of two early definitive studies are reproduced in tables 4.1 and 4.2. Table 4.1 shows the earliest age levels at which mastery of common consonants was achieved by 100% of the children studied by Davis (1938). In Table 4.2 Templin (1947) gives the age levels at which 75% of the children tested achieved mastery. Since the publication of the work of Davis and Templin, there has been little need to study the age levels at which phoneme mastery is attained. In recent years, research in phonological development has centered upon the ages at which phonemes emerge, not when they are mastered.

### Production of Phonemes

For many years, speech pathologists used tables such as those discussed above to determine whether articulation development was proceeding according to schedule. However, more recently they have focused on the child's production of phonemes and their relation to the words he or she is trying to produce. Even in the area of phonemics—the study of speech sounds—interest has shifted from the mere production of isolated phonemes to the acquisition of the distinctive features that make up the phonemes and to the acquisition of morphophonemic rules of syntax.

The child at the one-word stage of speech development creates sentences that have differing syntactic and semantic structures but that also preserve certain aspects of the phonemic segmental features within the words. For example, the child who says *ba-tuh* for *bottle* is preserving part of the consonant-vowel-consonant-vowel (C-V-C-V) segments of the word, and beyond that he or she is preserving the sequence of stop C + back V + stop C + back V (a statement in which C = consonant and V = vowel).

To account for what is preserved phonemically and what is not, Jakobson (1968) proposed the principle of maximum contrast and used it to explain the fact that infants' earliest utterances are usually *mama* and *papa*. These two utterances represent maximum contracts between +consonantal with −vocalic features (a consonant) and −consonantal with +vocalic (a vowel) and the lip sounds (/p/ and /m/). These consonants and vowels represent the largest degree of contrast, going from the anterior closure of the vocal mechanism to the opening of the posterior part. As further differentiations are made, additional phonemic features are acquired. For example, children

**TABLE 4.1. Earliest Age Level at Which Mastery was Attained by 100% of Children Tested**

| Age Levels in Years | | | | Phonemes | | | |
|---|---|---|---|---|---|---|---|
| 3.5 | m | p | b | w | h | | |
| 4.5 | n | t | d | ŋ | k | g | j |
| 5.5 | f | v | s* | z* | | | |
| 6.5 | ʃ | ʒ | l | θ | ð | | |
| 8.0 | r | hw | s | z | | | |

*/s/ and /z/ appear consistently at age 4.5 years but disappear when the anterior deciduous teeth are lost; they reappear after anterior dentition is complete.

Adapted from "The Speech Aspects of Reading Readiness" by I. Davis, 1938, *17th Yearbook of the Department of Elementary School Principals, 17,* pp. 282–289. Reprinted by permission.

**TABLE 4.2. Earliest Age Level of 75% Consonant Mastery**

| Age Levels in Years | | | | Phonemes | | | |
|---|---|---|---|---|---|---|---|
| 3.0 | m | n | n | p | f | h | w |
| 3.5 | j | | | | | | |
| 4.0 | b | d | k | g | r | | |
| 4.5 | s | ʃ | tʃ | | | | |
| 6.0 | t | l | v | θ | | | |
| 7.0 | ð | z | ʒ | dʒ | | | |

Adapted from *Certain Language Skills in Children* by M. Templin, Institute of Child Welfare Monograph Series No. 26, 1957, Minneapolis: University of Minnesota Press. Reprinted by permission.

can learn to distinguish between the oral feature of /p/ and the nasal feature of /m/, and they can begin to differentiate back vowels into their wide /a/ and narrow /i/ features.

## Sequence of Development

Based on the extensive work of researchers like Davis (1938) and Templin (1957) discussed earlier, there is a strong indication of a sequence in the development of differentiation of segmental features. This conclusion can be drawn simply because the data in tables 4.1 and 4.2 demonstrate that some phonemes are mastered before others. Menyuk (1968) analyzed these data and concluded that sounds that are +nasal, +grave, and +voice are mastered before those that are +diffuse, +continuant, and +strident.

With regard to the perceptual differentiation of segmental features, Edwards (1974), Lyamina and Gagua (1966), and Shvachkin (1966) all report that there is a sequence of development and that perceptual distinctions are made before productive distinctions. Whether the order of development is the same in perceptual and productive segments was investigated by Menyuk (1972) when she compared the results of her research on production substitutions with the research of Koenigsknecht and Lee on perceptual substitutions. The results indicate that the rank order for features preserved in perception and in production are not the same, although, as the reader may see in Table 4.3, there are similarities.

The earliest productive distinctions, that is, those made by children at age three, seem to be the following:

- oral versus nasal (*p, b, w* versus *m*)
- labial versus non-labial (*m, p, b* versus *n, t, d*)
- voiced versus non-voiced (*b, d* versus *p, t*)
- fricative versus stop (*f, v* versus *p, b*)
- lingual versus velar (*t, d, n* versus *k, g*)

**TABLE 4.3. Rank Order of Features Preserved in Perception and Production**

| Perception | Production |
|---|---|
| Nasality | Nasality |
| Voicing | Voicing |
| Continuancy | Stridency |
| Place | Continuancy |
| | Place |

From *The Development of Speech* (p. 26) by P. Menyuk, 1972, New York: Bobbs-Merrill. Reprinted by permission.

Children may distinguish these sounds earlier than others because these are the easiest ones to hear and because these are the perceptual distinctions that are easiest to translate into articulatory movements. The last sounds to be acquired (tables 4.1 and 4.2) are those in which the tongue must be moved to some position other than the normal rest position. Consider the differences in tongue movements for the production of /p/ or /b/ and for the production of /r/, /s/, or /ʃ/.

## The Morphophonemic Rules

In addition to acquiring the segmental features of phonology, the child at the same time is acquiring and developing certain sequential rules that relate to the syntax of his or her language—the morphophonemic rules. Newfield and Schlanger (1968) provide evidence that such rules are not fully mastered even by age 7. It appears, however, that it is the very specific rather than the general rules that are late in being learned. Some of the rules that are mastered late include:

- the past tense forms of strong verbs, such as *ring, rang*
- the /Iz/ versus the /s/ or /z/ ending for forming plurals or the third person singular
- The /Id/ versus the /t/ or /d/ ending for past tense

However, there is some evidence indicating that these rules are understood long before they are mastered in production (Menyuk & Klatt, 1968). As stated earlier, very young children are also able to differentiate between English and non-English clusters of consonants in reproducing non-English consonant clusters; they attempt to preserve the integrity of English rules, but they try to maintain the distinctive feature composition of the non-English clusters. Therefore, it may be concluded that these children are observing rules while also composing in segments. The reader probably knows from experience with young children that it is quite common to find them substituting /w/ for /r/ and /l/, as in *wabbit* for *rabbit* or *wady* for *lady*. These are perfectly acceptable English sound sequences and are not rejected by children making such substitutions.

In summary, children acquire and develop, in more or less identified sequence, the distinctive features that distinguish the phonemes of their language and the morphophonemic rules that govern the sequencing of the segments. In spite of the large body of research accrued in the past forty to fifty years, the study of the acquisition and development of the phonological system is still in its infancy. There has been a marked diminution of investigation in phonology; it is hoped that interest and activity will again increase in the not too distant future.

## SYNTACTICAL DEVELOPMENT

There is evidence that children in the early stages of speech development use single words as sentences, but the analysis of syntactic structures in development usually begins when the child has begun using two- and three-word sentences. Braine (1963) classifies the lexical items used by children in two categories: the open class and the pivot class. Generally, a small group of morphemes in the pivot class can occur in conjunction with many morphemes in the open class. McNeill (1970) assumes that the child generates sentences by selecting from the open class (O) in the case of one-word sentences or from either the open class twice (O,O) or the pivot and open class (P,O) in the case of longer utterances. A pivot grammar may describe a number of children's utterances, but, in general, it is too restrictive; children's language is hardly ever as simple as the pivot grammar concept would indicate (Bowerman, 1973). Many recent authors reject Chomsky's notion that there is a structure dependency of rules, that there are universal grammatical relations and categories (McNeill, 1966), or that grammatical rules are both analytic and productive. Instead, current theory and research indicate that the syntactic rules are semantic and that their source may be the child's cognitive structures.

This section on syntactical development encompasses structural development, Brown's stages of language development, and imitation. As the reader will note, there is considerable overlap among the various components of language, but the thread of syntax runs throughout the discussion.

### Structural Development

After children acquire base structure rules that define the subject-object relationship in sentences, they seem to acquire understanding of the concept that various sentence types can be generated by joining various elements such as negation + sentence, question + sentence, and so on. Under the heading of structural development, the emergence of complex and compound sentences is discussed. Menyuk (1971) provides a graphic explanation of the development of sentence types as shown in Table 4.4.

**Complex Sentences.** After the child has acquired true sentences, another equally important event in linguistic development occurs—the joining together of two simple sentences to form a complex sentence. If auxiliaries are excluded, one may say that any sentence containing two verbs represents two sentences in deep structure. The first complex sentences are often object noun-phrase complements and appear when the child has a mean length of utterance (MLU) of approximately 3.5 to 4.0 morphemes. In a

**TABLE 4.4. Stages in the Development of Declarative, Negative, Question, and Imperative Sentences**

| | A<br>Early | B<br>In Between | C<br>Later |
|---|---|---|---|
| Declarative | That box<br>Big boat<br>Rick go | That's box<br>That big boat<br>Rick going | That's a box<br>That's a big boat<br>Rick is going |
| Negative | No play<br>No a book<br>No fall down | I no play<br>That not book<br>(a) I not falling down<br>(b) I'm not fall down | I won't play<br>That's not a book<br>I'm not falling down |
| Question | See shoe?<br>Truck here?<br>Where baby? | Mommy see shoe?<br>Truck's here?<br>(a) Where baby is?<br>(b) Where's baby is? | Do you see the shoe?<br>Is the truck here?<br>Where's the baby? |
| Imperative | Want baby!<br><br><br>No touch!<br>Have it! | | I want the baby<br>or<br>Give me the baby!<br>Don't touch it!<br>Give it to me! |

From *The Acquisition and Development of Language* (p. 106) by P. Menyuk, 1971, Englewood Cliffs, NJ: Prentice-Hall. Reprinted by permission.

sentence with an object noun phrase complement, another full sentence can take the place of the object of the verb. For example:

- Watch me draw squares.
- I don't want you to watch TV.
- I saw you come in.

In these examples of children's language, the embedded sentence that is the object of the verb is present in the surface structure in its unembedded form. However, in adult English, complements appear to be quite different from simple sentences. "It annoys the neighbors for John to play basketball in the backyard" has as its object complement "John plays basketball." This is a type of complement that does not appear in child language until much later.

Sentences containing *wh-* clauses are a second type of complex sentence. The *wh-* clause allows one sentence to serve virtually any role in another sentence. The following are some examples of sentences with *wh-* clauses with embedded sentences shown in parentheses:

| | |
|---|---|
| • (Whoever did this) will pay for it | Subject |
| • He did (what he could) | Object |
| • I know (where he is) | Locative |

Relative clauses appear slightly later than the constructions noted above. They are related to *wh-* clauses, even though they are different from them. As indicated above, *wh-* clauses are embedded sentences used in a particular slot as a noun phrase. The relative clause, instead of being a noun phrase, modifies a noun phrase, as in "The man who came to dinner stayed a month," in which "The man who came to dinner" modifies and further specifies the subject of "the man stayed a month." Children first produce relative clauses to modify objects and predicate nominals and then later use them to modify subjects, as in the example given above. As a general rule, objects are modified before subjects whether the case is one of simple or complex modification.

**Compound Sentences.** Compound or conjoined sentences also begin to appear at this stage of development, but their mastery takes much longer. The first conjoined sentences produced by children seem to be simple groupings of two sentences without a conjuction, but shortly afterward the conjunction *and* makes its appearance. First sentences may be those like, "I see the book; you see the book." Later sentences would be like, "I was mad and I thought it was funny," in which the two sentences require the conjunction to establish the relationship between them.

## Brown's Stages of Language Development

Another way of looking at both syntactic and semantic language development in young children is provided by Brown (1973), who outlines five stages of development and discusses the first two stages in great detail. The following section deals with the results of Brown's extensive research into language development and the hypotheses he has derived from analyzing the results of that investigation.

Brown proposes five stages in language development, beginning with the first emergence of multiword utterances at Stage I and continuing through the development of complex sentences at Stage V. The stages are defined by increments of .5 to the mean length of utterance (MLU), but it should be remembered that there is a great deal of variation in length of utterance at any stage. Saying that a child has an MLU of 2.0 means that he or she may produce utterances that vary from one to six morphemes in length. However, children of comparable MLUs are as close to the same in language development as it is possible to find. Each stage is discussed below.

**Stage I.** Brown characterizes children's Stage I speech in several ways. The first aspect of construction he calls relations or roles within the simple sentence. More descriptively, he discusses Stage I as a time of telegraphic speech and the pivot grammar. Telegraphic speech is exactly what the term seems to mean: an absence of the small functional words, such as prepositions, articles, conjunctions, auxiliary verbs, and so on. Those words that we leave out of telegrams are omitted from the speech of Stage I children.

The pivot grammar was discussed briefly in the previous section of this chapter. However, more explanation of the Stage I construction is warranted. In the production by a child of a single sentence, "Mommy sock," Bloom (1970) concludes that the context in which the utterance is made determines the meaning of the sentence. Viewed contextually, the sentence is actually at least two different sentences. In one sentence, *Mommy* is a possessive modifier of sock in *Mommy's sock,* and in the second, *Mommy* is the agent of the sentence and *sock* is the object. A pivot grammar could not distinguish between the two sentences, but it is clear that the relationship between *Mommy* and *sock* differs in the two. There are other common semantic relationships in Stage I sentences, as shown in Table 4.5. As with Bloom's *Mommy sock* sentence, it is necessary to know the context to determine the semantic relationship.

Brown has extended further the explanation of semantic relations in the Stage I sentence by defining and exemplifying some of the semantic roles played by noun phrases in simple sentences. Table 4.6, which demonstrates some of the roles, is taken from *A First Language* (Brown, 1973).

The essential points to be remembered in the analysis of a language sample with regard to Stage I language behavior are that (a) it is marked by a reliance on telegraphic speech, (b) the semantic relationships between words in sentences are as shown in Table 4.5, and (c) the noun phrases in simple sentences may play a number of roles as described in Table 4.6. All of this behavior is typical of the Stage I child whose MLU is 1.01 to 1.99 morphemes.

**Stage II.** The child with an MLU of 2.00 to 2.49 is said to be in Stage II of language development—a stage referred to by Brown (1973) as a stage of modulating meaning within the simple sentence. In English, modulations are defined as structures such as the inflection of the noun for plurality; inflection of the verb for tense; provision of the copula *be*; provision of definite and indefinite articles that are used to mark a referent; and some prepositions like *in* and *on* that are used to further specify locations suggested by word order alone. Brown selected 14 grammatical morphemes

**TABLE 4.5. Semantic Relations in Stage I Sentences**

| Semantic Relation | Form | Example |
|---|---|---|
| 1. Nomination | that + N | that book |
| 2. Notice | hi + N | hi belt |
| 3. Recurrence | more + N, 'nother + N | more milk |
| 4. Nonexistence | allgone + N, no more + N | allgone rattle |
| 5. Attributive | Adj + N | big train |
| 6. Possessive | N + N | mommy lunch |
| 7. Locative | N + N | sweater chair |
| 8. Locative | V + N | walk street |
| 9. Agent-Action | N + V | Eve read |
| 10. Agent-Object | N + N | Mommy sock |
| 11. Action-Object | V + N | put book |

Adapted from *Psycholinguistics* (p. 220) by R. Brown, 1970, New York: Free Press, a Division of Macmillan. Reprinted by permission.

for study, as shown in Table 4.7. These morphemes are almost totally missing from Stage I; in Stage II they begin to appear, but even by Stage V some children have not yet reached the 90% mastery level on some morphemes. The inflections of meaning occur in a lengthy development—a property that English may share with other languages. The modulations shown in Table 4.7 do not constitute an exhaustive list for English; Brown selected only forms for which it is possible to identify contexts in which the form is obligatory.

**Stage III.** In stages I and II, Brown describes the major semantic relations and development of inflections (modulations) in what are essentially declarative and affirmative simple sentences. In Stage III other sentence modalities are considered: *yes-no* interrogatives, constituent interrogatives, imperatives, and negatives. Brown uses the sentence, "Mr. Smith cut the rope with a knife," to demonstrate that it can be transformed into an interrogative that requires a *yes* response if assenting or a *no* if dissenting. The interrogative transformation becomes, "Did Mr. Smith cut the rope with a knife?" None of the semantic relations nor modulations discussed under Stage II are altered in this transformation, although the reader should note that the

**TABLE 4.6. Some Semantic Roles Played by Noun Phrases in Simple Sentences**

| Role | Definition | Examples |
|---|---|---|
| Agent | Someone or something that causes or instigates an action or process. Usually animate but not always, an agent must be perceived to have its own motivating force. | *Harriet* sang.<br>*The men* laughed.<br>*The wind* ripped the curtains. |
| Patient | Someone or something either in a given state or suffering a change | *The wood* is dry.<br>He cut *the wood.* |
| Experiencer | Someone having a given experience or mental disposition | *Tom* saw the snake.<br>*Tom* wanted a drink. |
| Beneficiary | Someone who profits from a state or process, including possession | *Mary* has a convertible.<br>This is *Mary's* car.<br>Tom bought *Mary* a car. |
| Instrument | Something that plays a role in bringing about a process or action but which is not the instigator; it is used by an agent | Tom opened the door with *a key.*<br>Tom used *his knife* to open the box. |
| Location | The place or locus of a state, action, or process | The spoon is in *the drawer.*<br>Tom sat in *the chair.* |
| Complement | The verb names an action that brings something into existence. The complement, on a more or less specific level, completes the verb. This use of the word "complement" is not, incidentally, its most common use in linguistics. | Mary sang *a song.*<br>John played *checkers.* |

From *A First Language: The Early Stages* (p. 8) by R. Brown, 1973, Cambridge, MA: Harvard University Press. Reprinted by permission.

## TABLE 4.7. The Acquisition of 14 English Grammatical Morphemes

| Morpheme | Order of Acquisition | Semantic Description | Example |
|---|---|---|---|
| present progressive | 1 | temporary duration | The dog *is barking.* |
| on | 2.5 | support | The book is *on* the table. |
| in | 2.5 | containment | The candy is *in* the box. |
| plural | 4 | more than one | The boy*s* are here. |
| past irregular | 5 | earlierness | He *came.* |
| possessive | 6 | ownership | The man*'s* hat is black. |
| uncontractible copula | 7 | identity<br>membership<br>attribute possession<br>location | *These are* white.<br>*These are* cocker spaniels.<br>The dogs *are* white.<br>Here it *is.* |
| Articles | 8 | specific<br>nonspecific | *The* horse is brown.<br>I have *a* box. |
| past regular | 9 | earlierness | They *walked* to town. |
| third person singular regular | 10 | tense, number (often is redundant) | The boy *walks.* |
| third person singular irregular | 11 | tense, number | The boy *has* a hat. |
| uncontractible auxiliary | 12 | temporary duration<br>earlierness | *These are* going on the shelf.<br>*They were* going to town. |
| contractible copula | 13 | identity<br>membership<br>attribute possession<br>location | *He's* John.<br>*Daddy's* a man.<br>The *book's* blue.<br>*Mary's* at home. |
| contractible auxiliary | 14 | temporary duration<br>earlierness | *He's* talked too long.<br>*He'd* talked too long. |

From *A First Language: The Early Stages* (p. 31) by R. Brown, 1973, Cambridge, MA: Harvard University Press. Reprinted by permission.

auxiliary *do* had to be supplied and marked for past tense—*did*. In addition, there are tag questions such as, "You're going, aren't you?" that are also requests for confirmation through a *yes-no* response. However, tag questions are very late in the course of development, and some Stage V children still have not acquired them.

Another form of interrogative sentence that makes its appearance in Stage III is the question requesting that a constituent be named—or more commonly, the *wh-* question. These are termed *wh-* questions, because in almost all instances the question is initiated by *who, whose, what, where, when, why,* or *how* (e.g., "Who will take out the trash?"). The constituent required in the response to the question is a subject noun: "X will take out the trash."

In Stage III the negative sentence, as opposed to the syntactic expression of negation (No!), begins to appear. Bloom (1970) distinguishes three types of negation: nonexistence, rejection, and denial. Nonexistence of a referent can be expressed as, "There isn't any milk," ordinarily meaning that there was some milk but now there is not. Rejection is exemplified in a sentence such as, "I don't want any milk," or "No more milk." Finally, there is the negative sentence that denies the truth of some proposition, such as, "Texas is not part of the U.S."

Imperative sentences are those in which the speaker asks, demands, insists, and so on, that something occur. In English, we have no difficulty identifying the imperative, because it is usually expressed without a subject and begins only with the uninflected verb, as in, "Pass the butter," "Give me a hand," and so on. The imperative is considered a characteristic of Stage III but is present even in Stage I children. On purely linguistic grounds, imperatives are almost impossible to identify, because the Stage I child so often produces subjectless sentences. Therefore, it is only from context that we know the child is expressing an imperative. By Stage III the child will use subjects in sentences, and we can easily recognize the imperative when it appears.

Many of the transformations of Stage III make their initial, unstructured appearance as far back as Stage I, but they become truly identifiable only in Stage III. Furthermore, the elaboration of the transformations occurs after Stage III and even past Stage IV. The most acceptable method of categorizing a child as being in Stage III is to apply the MLU method: If the child's MLU is 2.50 to 2.99 morphemes, we may say that he or she is in Stage III.

**Stage IV.** Three varieties of embedded sentences begin to appear in Stage IV: object noun phrase complements, indirect or embedded *wh-* questions, and relative clauses. Remember that we are discussing a child with a predicted chronological age of only 3.0 to perhaps 3.5 years and that the discussion of embedded sentences does not apply in its fullest sophistication to such a young child. Rather, one sees the early beginnings of embedding in Stage IV, and the full elaboration of embedding may not be observed in many adults.

The easiest embeddings to recognize are the object noun phrase complements which take the form of, "I hope I don't hurt it," "I think it's the wrong way," and other sentences recorded by Brown (1973). These were early productions of the children he observed. In these sentences, one can see that with certain transitive verbs, (e.g., *think, know, guess, tell, hope,* and *mean*), a simple intact sentence may take the place of a simple noun object and play the role of a noun. It is much more difficult to recognize the simple sentence, "Mary plays the piano," in the more complex sentence, "It bothers the neighbors for Mary to play the piano," and yet the same kind of complement is used in the two sentences.

The second type of embedding involves the use of *wh-* questions. Brown (1973) recorded a number of these sentences, a few of which are:

> Whoever broke this must fix it.
> When I get big I can lift you up.
> Mary sang what I like to hear. (p. 22)

These sentences are indirect (or embedded) *wh-* questions in which the *wh-* word plays the role of the object or some other role.

A classically constructed sentence with a relative clause is, "The man who came to dinner stayed a month," in which there are two propositions made about the same noun phrase. Because a relative pronoun (e.g., *who, whom, which*) may replace a noun phrase, it is not always apparent that there are two propositions.

**Stage V.** Stage V is marked by an MLU of 4.00 to 4.49 morphemes with a predicted chronological age of 43.4 to 46.6 months, as may be seen in Table 4.8. It is a stage titled by Brown as "coordination of simple sentences and propositional relations." Early examples of coordinated simple sentences are, "I have one and you have one," "John plays and Mary plays," and so on. Each of the simple sentences is complete and can stand alone, but it usually demonstrates a continuity of thought. The sentence, "I am an educator and Mary has a cat," is not patently ungrammatic, but it violates the underlying semantic relationships that we expect in coordinated sentences. As language develops, children eliminate the redundancy in the sentences given above and instead replace them with, "You and I have one," or, "John and Mary play."

Brown (1973) summarizes the five stages as follows:

> In summary five major processes of sentence construction have been described in both semantic and syntactic terms . . . They are:
>
> 1. Semantic roles such as agent, patient, instrument, locative, etc., in simple sentences expressed by linear order, syntactic relations, prepositions or postpositions.
>
> 2. Semantic modulations such as number, specificity, tense, aspect, mood, etc., expressed by inflections or free forms belonging to small closed classes.
>
> 3. Modalities of the simple sentence: *yes-no* interrogation, request for specification of a constituent, negation, imperative.
>
> 4. Embedding of one simple sentence as a grammatical constituent or in a semantic role in another including all the roles of 1, all the constituents which one may ask to be specified in 3.

5. Coordination of full sentences or of partially identical and partially distinct (but structurally matched) sentences with deletion of one representation of the identical stretches. The coordinated sentences appear with connector words that approximate in meaning to relations of propositional logic. (p. 32)

## Imitation

So far we have discussed only the spontaneous production of language, but a great deal of research effort has been spent on investigating the imitation performance of children. Two types of imitation have been studied: spontaneous imitation (in which the child imitates an adult's production without being cued) and elicited imitation (in which an adult asks the child to imitate him). In general, three conclusions can be drawn from the studies done by Ervin (1964), Kemp and Dale (1973), and Bloom, Hood, and Lightbown (1974). These studies are prototypical of many others that have been done.

First, imitations have essentially the same structure as the child's free speech no matter how complicated the stimulus is. Second, the imitations may even be simpler in structure than the child's free speech. Third, children may imitate new words that have not occurred in their free speech yet may *not* imitate words that are in their everyday productive vocabulary. This last point, that children may not imitate words or structures that are in their spontaneous speech, is a particularly interesting one. Bloom (1974) hypothesizes that in spontaneous speech, the child is talking about the present—the here and now—and that this temporal contextual support plays an important role in the formulation of sentences. Without this support, children do not seem to be able to produce utterances in imitation that they have produced spontaneously the day before.

In regard to syntactic development, another aspect should be discussed, that of comprehension. If a child does not spontaneously produce a particular structure, such as plurals, and does not imitate plural words, can one be sure that the concept of plurality is not a part of the child's competence? It does seem that children comprehend language long before they produce it, but sometimes their apparent ability to comprehend is deceiving. Consider that when a child hears a word, he or she has several clues to its meaning: his or her own general knowledge of the world, the nonlinguistic context in which the word occurs, the linguistic context, and the child's knowledge of words and syntactic structures. When any of us hears a word, we call upon these clues. A child may respond appropriately to the command, "Come here," only because of minimal gestural cues. He or she may respond to, "Give it to daddy," because of the linguistic context and because it is the child's mother speaking.

The first systematic attempt to investigate and compare imitation, comprehension, and production was made by Fraser, Bellugi, and Brown (1963).

## TABLE 4.8. Predicted Chronological Ages and Age Ranges Within One Standard Deviation of the Predicted Value for Each MLU

| Brown's stage | MLU | Predicted chronological age[a] | Predicted age ±1 SD[b] (middle 68%) |
|---|---|---|---|
| Early Stage I | 1.01 | 19.1 | 16.4–21.8 |
| MLU = 1.01–1.49 | 1.10 | 19.8 | 17.1–22.5 |
| | 1.20 | 20.6 | 17.9–23.3 |
| | 1.30 | 21.4 | 18.7–24.1 |
| | 1.40 | 22.2 | 19.5–24.9 |
| | 1.50 | 23.0 | 18.5–27.5 |
| Late Stage I | 1.60 | 23.8 | 19.3–28.3 |
| MLU = 1.50–1.99 | 1.70 | 24.6 | 20.1–29.1 |
| | 1.80 | 25.3 | 20.8–29.8 |
| | 1.90 | 26.1 | 21.6–30.6 |
| | 2.00 | 26.9 | 21.5–32.3 |
| Stage II | 2.10 | 27.7 | 22.3–33.1 |
| MLU = 2.00–2.49 | 2.20 | 28.5 | 23.1–33.9 |
| | 2.30 | 29.3 | 23.9–34.7 |
| | 2.40 | 30.1 | 24.7–35.5 |
| | 2.50 | 30.8 | 23.9–37.7 |
| Stage III | 2.60 | 31.6 | 24.7–38.5 |
| MLU = 2.50–2.99 | 2.70 | 32.4 | 25.5–39.3 |
| | 2.80 | 33.2 | 26.3–40.1 |
| | 2.90 | 34.0 | 27.1–40.9 |
| | 3.00 | 34.8 | 28.0–41.6 |
| Early Stage IV | 3.10 | 35.6 | 28.8–42.4 |
| MLU = 3.00–3.49 | 3.20 | 36.3 | 29.5–43.1 |
| | 3.30 | 37.1 | 30.3–43.9 |
| | 3.40 | 37.9 | 31.1–44.7 |
| | 3.50 | 38.7 | 30.8–46.6 |
| Late Stage IV– | 3.60 | 39.5 | 31.6–47.4 |
| Early Stage V | 3.70 | 40.3 | 32.4–48.2 |
| MLU = 3.50–3.99 | 3.80 | 41.1 | 33.2–49.0 |
| | 3.90 | 41.8 | 33.9–49.7 |
| | 4.00 | 42.6 | 36.7–48.5 |

**TABLE 4.8.** continued

| Brown's stage | MLU | Predicted chronological age[a] | Predicted age ±1 SD[b] (middle 68%) |
|---|---|---|---|
| Late Stage V | 4.10 | 43.4 | 37.5–49.3 |
| MLU = 4.00–4.49 | 4.20 | 44.2 | 38.3–50.1 |
| | 4.30 | 45.0 | 39.1–50.9 |
| | 4.40 | 45.8 | 39.9–51.7 |
| | 4.50 | 46.6 | 40.3–52.9 |
| Post Stage V | 4.60 | 47.3 | 41.0–53.6 |
| MLU = 4.50+ | 4.70 | 48.2 | 41.9–54.5 |
| | 4.80 | 48.9 | 42.6–55.2 |
| | 4.90 | 49.7 | 43.4–56.0 |
| | 5.00 | 50.5 | 42.1–58.9 |
| | 5.10 | 51.3 | 42.9–59.7 |
| | 5.20 | 52.1 | 43.7–60.5 |
| | 5.30 | 52.8 | 44.4–61.2 |
| | 5.40 | 53.6 | 45.2–62.0 |
| | 5.50 | 54.4 | 46.0–62.8 |
| | 5.60 | 55.2 | 46.8–63.6 |
| | 5.70 | 56.0 | 47.6–64.4 |
| | 5.80 | 56.8 | 48.4–65.2 |
| | 5.90 | 57.5 | 49.1–65.9 |
| | 6.00 | 58.3 | 49.9–66.7 |

[a]Age is predicted from the equation Age (in months) = 11.199 + 7.857 (MLU)
[b]Computed from obtained standard deviations

From *Assessing Language Production in Children: Experimental Procedures* (p. 26) by J. Miller, 1981, Austin, TX: PRO-ED. Reprinted by permission

Using the Imitation–Comprehension–Production Test (ICP), they combined pairs of sentences that differed in only one aspect, such as plurality, and asked children to imitate the sentences, to point to the picture that correctly depicted the sentences, and to produce a correct sentence when shown a picture. For the ten pairs of sentences, the results were remarkably clear-cut and consistent. The children scored highest on the imitation task, second highest on the comprehension section, and lowest on production. In fact, this pattern occurred in almost all of the children tested. The children ranged in age from 37 to 43 months. The study was so intriguing that it was replicated by Lovell and Dixon (1967) with children aged 2 to 6 years and with retarded 6 and 7 year olds. Their results were the same as those of the earlier study, with the addition of the finding that scores increased with age and with intellectual level.

The results of studies mentioned above do not necessarily refute the findings of Bloom and others; the children were tested on elicited and not spontaneous imitations. However, other problems with the ICP type of studies have been noted by Baird (1972) and Fernald (1972).

After the age of 5 or 6 years, syntactic development—at least in production—appears to approximate adult language quite closely, with a few common difficulties that can be noted. These problems include subject-verb agreement, case endings on personal pronouns, acquisition of the irregular past tense, and acquisition of perfect forms. As the reader can see, these are relatively minor matters of development. For all purposes one may say that the basic syntactic structure of the majority of the older child's sentences is the same as that of adult grammar, with the one notable exception of complex sentences. For information on later syntactic development with regard to specific structures, the reader may refer to Chomsky (1968), Cromer (1970), Kessel (1970), and Cambon and Sinclair (1974).

## SEMANTIC AND PRAGMATIC DEVELOPMENT

During the past ten years or so, many studies have addressed themselves to the relationship between cognitive and linguistic development (Bates, Camaioni, & Volterra, 1975; Blank, 1974, 1975; Bowerman, 1976, 1977; Cromer, 1981; Duchan, 1983; Morehead & Morehead, 1974; Schlesinger, 1974, 1977; Sinclair-de-Zwart, 1969; Wells, 1975). No attempt will be made to summarize the work and/or positions of all these authors; suffice it to say there seem to be three major propositions: (a) Cognitive development precedes language development; (b) cognition and language develop in a parallel but noncausally related fashion; and (c) some unidentified "deeper" structures account for both cognitive and language development. At present, the state of the field is one in which one author supposes and another disposes; however, all seem to be very polite to one another at this juncture, probably because it is anyone's guess as to who is correct. Simply, the results are not yet in.

Setting aside the above issues, we will concentrate on a somewhat demographic view of semantic and pragmatic development. Again, emphasis will be on *what* rather than *how* or *why*. It is convenient to follow Katz and Langendown (1976) in relating pragmatics to the study of meaning and making a distinction between grammatical meaning and utterance meaning. They equate pragmatics with semantic performance and indicate that pragmatics may be viewed as the performance aspect of the semantic component of grammar.

## Lexical Growth

Semantic development has been reviewed by most authors in terms of lexical growth—the acquisition of words that have meaning to the child. Bloom (1973) originally contended that single words might be used by the child to express an entire sentence and that the child omitted the rest of the words because of limited performance factors such as memory span or breath control. Bloom also wrote that the single words used by the child were gross approximations of the adult word and that by adding semantic features, the child could come closer and closer to the dictionary meaning of the word. Within this notion are two well-known facts related to the development of word meaning: overextension and underextension (or overlap). Overextension refers to word meanings that are overgeneralized (e.g., the use of *dog* to refer to all animals). On the other hand, underextensions are word meanings that are too specific (e.g., *dog* used to refer only to the family pet).

From the literature, it appears that overextension is the more common failing of children developing language, but there are notable exceptions. Seldom are proper names overgeneralized, and diaries of children's language development are replete with underextensions. Therefore, it is probably impossible to say which failure is the more common. One serious problem with H. Clark's (1970) theory is her failure to account for the occurrence of underextensions.

## Variable Word Meanings

Briefly, some of the research dealing with the development of the meaning of specific terms will be discussed. The terms *more* and *less* were studied in 3 year olds by Donaldson and Balfour (1968) and Palermo (1973), all of whom found that the terms were treated generally as synonyms. The children reacted as if they knew that the terms referred to quantity, but they did not distinguish between them.

Dimensional terms (e.g., *big, little, long, short, thick, thin*) have been extensively explored by Donaldson and Wales (1970), H. Clark (1970), E. Clark (1972), Maratsos (1973), and Eilers, Oller, and Ellington (1974). Some of the findings are: (a) Fewer errors were recorded for the *big/little* contrast than for any of the others and (b) there were fewer on *long/short* than on *wide/narrow,* indicating a developmental trend from general to specific terms. However, for all three contrasts, correct responses occurred most frequently on the negative item in the pair—that is, *little, short,* and *narrow.* Maratsos' findings suggest a three-stage development in the meanings of *big* and *long,* as follows:

- About age 3: *big* refers to global (overall size, and *long* refers to only one dimension

- About age 4–5: *long* is still interpreted correctly, but now *big* is treated as synonymous with *long*, particularly with reference to height
- About age 5+: the two terms are again distinguished correctly

Apparently, learning the meanings of words is not merely a matter of the child attending to the adult language features of the word; in fact, quite different features may be used during language development.

In addition to the above research, various authors have investigated causality and verbs, verbs of possession and transfer, color names, and many other structures. Some good reviews can be found in Bloom (1973), Hayes (1970), John and Moskovitch (1970), Moore (1973), and Slobin (1973).

## SUMMARY

Language development was discussed in this chapter with reference to the young child's development of phonological, syntactic, and semantic structures and rules. In addition, a fairly lengthy review of the stages of language development according to Brown (1973) was presented because of its marked relevance to the analysis of language samples. As stated in the beginning of the chapter, the discussion of development was felt to be necessary, because the orientation to assessment presented throughout the text is developmental. Without a thorough grounding in language development, the clinician will have great difficulty in adopting such an approach. Although the discussion is brief in relation to the body of knowledge regarding language development, the clinician should be able to extend his or her knowledge by pursuing some of the references given.

## REFERENCES

Baird, R. (1972). On the role of chance in Imitation–Comprehension–Production Test results. *Journal of Verbal Learning and Verbal Behavior, 11,* 474–477.

Bates, E., Camaioni, L., & Volterra, V. (1975). The acquisition of performatives prior to speech. *Merrill-Palmer Quarterly, 21,* 205–226.

Blank, M. (1974). Cognitive functions of language in the preschool years. *Developmental Psychology, 10,* 229–245.

Blank, M. (1975). Mastering the intangible through language. In D. Aaronson & R. Rieber (Eds.), *Developmental psycholinguistics and communication disorders* (pp. 234–249). New York: New York Academy of Sciences.

Bloom, L. (1970). *Language development: Form and function in emerging grammars.* Cambridge, MA: MIT Press.

Bloom, L. (1973). *One word at a time.* The Hague: Mouton.

Bloom, L. (1974). Talking, understanding, and thinking. In R. Schiefelbusch & L. Lloyd (Eds.), *Language perspectives: Acquisition, retardation, and intervention* (pp. 285–311). Austin, TX: PRO-ED.

Bloom, L., Hood, L., & Lightbown, P. (1974). Imitation in language development. *Cognitive Psychology, 6,* 380–420.

Bowerman, M. (1973). Structural relationships in children's utterances: Syntactic or semantic? In I. E. Moore (Ed.), *Cognitive development and the acquisition of language* (pp. 346–378). New York: Academic Press.

Bowerman, M. (1976). Semantic factors in the acquisition of rules for word use and sentence construction. In D. Morehead & A. Morehead (Eds.), *Directions in normal and deficient child language* (pp. 99–179). Austin, TX: PRO-ED.

Bowerman, M. (1977). The acquisition of rules governing "possible lexical items": Evidence from spontaneous speech errors. Stanford University Department of Linguistics, *Papers/Reports on Child Language Development, 13,* 148–156.

Braine, M. (1963). The ontogeny of English phrase structure: The first phrase. *Language, 39,* 1–14.

Brown, R. (1973). *A first language: The early stages.* Cambridge, MA: Harvard University Press.

Cambon, J., & Sinclair, H. (1974). Relations between syntax and semantics: Are they "easy to see?" *British Journal of Psychology, 65,* 133–140.

Chomsky, C. (1968). *The acquisition of syntax in children from 5 to 10.* Cambridge, MA: MIT Press.

Chomsky, N. (1957). *Syntactic structures.* The Hague: Mouton.

Chomsky, N. (1968). *Language and mind.* New York: Harcourt, Brace & World.

Clark, E. (1972). On the child's acquisition of antonyms in two semantic fields. *Journal of Verbal Learning and Verbal Behavior, 11,* 750–758.

Clark, E. (1973). What's in a word? On the child's acquisition of semantics in his first language. In T. E. Moore (Ed.), *Cognitive development and the acquisition of language* (pp. 65–110). New York: Academic Press.

Clark, H. (1970). The primitive nature of children's relational concepts. In J. Hayes (Ed.), *Cognition and the development of language* (pp. 324–333). New York: John Wiley.

Cromer, R. (1970). Children are nice to understand: Surface structure clues for the recovery of a deep structure. *British Journal of Psychology, 61,* 397–408.

Cromer, R. (1981). Reconceptualizing language acquisition and cognitive development. In R. Schiefelbusch & D. Bricker (Eds.), *Early language: Acquisition and intervention* (pp. 51–138). Austin, TX: PRO-ED.

Davis, I. (1938). The speech aspects of reading readiness. *17th Yearbook of the Department of Elementary School Principals, 17,* 282–289.

Donaldson, M., & Balfour, G. (1968). Less is more: A study of language comprehension in children. *British Journal of Psychology, 59,* 461–472.

Donaldson, M., & Wales, R. (1970). On the acquisition of some relational terms. In J. Hayes (Ed.), *Cognition and the development of language* (pp. 112–123). New York: John Wiley.

Duchan, J. (1983). Language processing and geodesic domes. In T. Gallagher & C. Prutting (Eds.), *Pragmatic assessment and intervention issues* (pp. 83–101). College-Hill Press.

Edwards, M. (1974). Perception and production in child phonology: The testing of four hypotheses. *Journal of Child Language, 1,* 205–219.

Eilers, R., Oller, D., & Ellington, J. (1974). The acquisition of word meaning for dimensional adjectives: The long and short of it. *Journal of Child Language, 1,* 195–204.

Ervin, S. (1964). Imitation and structural change in children's language. In E. Lenneberg (Ed.), *New directions in the study of language* (pp. 163–189). Cambridge, MA: MIT Press.

Fernald, C. (1972). Control of grammar in imitation, comprehension, and production: Problems of replication. *Journal of Verbal Learning and Verbal Behavior, 11,* 606–613.

Fraser, C., Bellugi, U., & Brown, R. (1963). Control of grammar in imitation, comprehension, and production. *Journal of Verbal Learning and Verbal Behavior, 2,* 121–135.

Hayes, J. (Ed.). (1970). *Cognition and the development of language.* New York: John Wiley.

Irwin, O. (1947). Infant speech: Consonantal sounds according to place of articulation. *Journal of Speech Disorders, 12,* 187–201.

Irwin, O. (1948). Infant speech: Development of vowel sounds. *Journal of Speech and Hearing Disorders, 13,* 31–34.

John, V., & Moskovitch, S. (1970). Language acquisition and development in early childhood. In A. Marckwardt (Ed.), *Linguistics in school programs* (pp. 167–214). Chicago: National Society for the Study of Education.

Katz, J., & Langendoen, D. (1976). Pragmatics and presuppositions. *Language, 52,* 1917.

Kemp, J., & Dale, P. (1973, March). Spontaneous imitation and free speech: A grammatical comparison. Paper presented to the Society for Research in Child Development, Philadelphia.

Kessel, F. (1970). The role of syntax in children's comprehension from ages six to ten. *Monographs of the Society for Research in Child Development, 35,* No. 6 (Serial No. 139).

Lovell, K., & Dixon, E. (1967). The growth of the control of grammar in imitation, comprehension, and production. *Journal of Child Psychology and Psychiatry, 8,* 31–39.

Lyamina, G. M., & Gagua, N. I. (1966). On the formation of the correct pronunciation of words in children from 1½ to 3 years of life. In F. Smith & G. A. Miller (Eds.), *The genesis of language* (pp. 374–375). Cambridge, MA: MIT Press.

McNeill, D. (1966). Developmental psycholinguistics. In F. Smith & G. Miller (Eds.), *The genesis of language* (pp. 15–84). Cambridge, MA: MIT Press.

McNeill, D. (1970). *The acquisition of language: The study of developmental psycholinguistics.* New York: Harper and Row.

Maratsos, M. (1973). Decrease in the understanding of the word "big" in preschool children. *Child Development, 44,* 747–752.

Menyuk, P. (1968). The role of distinctive features in children's acquisition of phonology. *Journal of Speech and Hearing Research, 11,* 138–146.

Menyuk, P. (1971). *The acquisition and development of language.* Englewood Cliffs, NJ: Prentice-Hall.

Menyuk, P. (1972). *The development of speech.* New York: Bobbs-Merrill.

Menyuk, P., & Klatt, D. (1968). A child's production of initial consonant clusters. *Quarterly Progress Reports of the Research Laboratory of Electonics, MIT, 91,* 205–213.

Moore, T. (1973). *Cognitive development and the acquisition of language.* New York: Academic Press.

Morehead, D., & Morehead, A. (1974). From signal to sign: A Piagetian view of thought and language during the first two years. In R. Schiefelbusch & L. Lloyd (Eds.), *Language perspectives: Acquisition, retardation, and intervention* (pp. 153–190). Austin, TX: PRO-ED.

Newfield, M., & Schlanger, B. (1968). The acquisition of English morphology by normal and educable mentally retarded children. *Journal of Speech and Hearing Research, 11,* 693–706.

Palermo, D. S. (1973). More about less: A study of language comprehension. *Journal of Verbal Learning and Verbal Behavior, 13,* 211–221.

Schlesinger, I. (1974). Relational concepts underlying language. In R. Schiefelbusch & L. Lloyd (Eds.), *Language perspectives: Acquisition, retardation, and intervention* (pp. 129–151). Austin, TX: PRO-ED.

Schlesinger, I. (1977). The role of cognitive development and linguistic input in language acquisition. *Journal of Child Language, 4,* 153–169.

Shvachkin, N. (1966). Development of phonemic speech perception in early childhood. Abstracted by D. Slobin. In F. Smith & G. Miller (Eds.), *The genesis of language* (pp. 381–382). Cambridge, MA: MIT Press.

Sinclair-de-Zwart, H. (1969). Developmental psycholinguistics. In D. Elkind & J. Flavell (Eds.), *Studies in cognitive development* (pp. 315–366). New York: Oxford University Press.

Slobin, D. (1973). Cognitive prerequisites for the development of grammar. In C. Ferguson & D. Slobin (Eds.), *Studies of child language development* (pp. 183–186). New York: Rinehart, Holt, and Winston.

Templin, M. (1957). *Certain language skills in children.* Institute of Child Welfare Monograph Series, No. 26. Minneapolis: University of Minnesota Press.

Wells, G. (1975). Interpersonal communication and the development of language. Paper presented at the Third International Child Language Symposium, London, September.

# 5 / THE ASSESSMENT PROCEDURES

The present chapter deals with the assessment and description of oral language delay or disorder in children who may have a variety of other handicapping conditions. As indicated in the preface, the philosophy of assessment reflected in this text centers around the need to describe the child's comprehension and production of language through a developmental investigation of the processes of language. The chapter is presented in three main sections: standardized measures of oral language, the language sample, and other assessment procedures. The section on standardized measures of oral language deals briefly with a few of the more commonly used instruments, because they are considered the best vehicle for identifying children with significant linguistic discrepancies. The second section describes one of the oldest techniques for assessing oral language production—the collecting and analyzing of a language sample. In the third section, which is by far the longest of the three, a number of informal assessment strategies are discussed.

## STANDARDIZED MEASURES OF ORAL LANGUAGE

A variety of frequently used standardized and often normed measures of oral language are on the commercial market. Some of these measures assess only one dimension of language, such as articulation or syntax; others purport to assess almost all parameters of spoken language. In the following section, two general types of tests are discussed: (a) measures of only phonology and (b) measures that assess syntax, semantics, and, sometimes, articulation.

## Tests of Phonology

In this section phonological tests of both reception and production are discussed. Phonological reception may be considered synonymous with speech sound discrimination, while phonological production is discussed in terms of articulatory performance. The tests reviewed in this section are at least partially standardized in that specific instructions are provided for administration and scoring. There is a great deal of latitude permitted in the interpretation of the scores, and the reader will find that there are no exact norms.

**Tests of Speech Sound Discrimination.** Most investigators have found a relationship between speech sound discrimination and articulatory proficiency that they feel indicates the following: (a) Children's speech sound discrimination ability improves as they grow older, at least during the period between the ages of 3 and 8 years: and (b) children who have articulation deficits also tend to have poor speech sound discrimination. Clinicians usually assess articulation defective children in speech sound discrimination as a precursor to teaching them to hear the differences among sounds in the auditory training phase of therapy. Only two tests of speech sound discrimination are discussed, because there is a marked similarity among all such tests.

*Auditory Discrimination Test.* The *Auditory Discrimination Test* (Wepman, 1958) is the prototype for many discrimination tests, both standardized and nonstandardized. It was constructed for children between the ages of 5 to 8 years and consists of 40 word pairs, such as *sake/shake.* The test is administered by having the child turn his or her back to the examiner and indicating whether the two words produced by the examiner are the same or different. The test incorporates a validity check to determine whether the child understands the task and is able to cooperate in taking it. As would be expected, it is necessary to determine whether the child understands the concepts of *same* and *different* before administering a test like this. Broadly stated age norms are provided.

*Language Related Tests of Speech-Sound Discrimination (LTSD).* The LTSD (Bryen, 1974) was developed as a means of determining whether a child has adequate speech sound discrimination in standard English, black English, and Spanish. The test consists of three different forms, one in each language area, and has 35 items per form. It is appropriate for children 6 to 12 years old. The LTSD uses the Wepman paradigm in which the first word is presented, followed by a second word, which is the same as the first or which differs in only one phoneme. The child responds by indicating whether the two words are the same or different.

The test can serve several purposes. First, information can be obtained as to how children are developing phonologically in their own spoken language, and second, one can determine how well children are developing in standard English regardless of the language they use. Statistical data provided indicate that the age-related construct validity of the LTSD is partially supported and that the test-retest reliability coefficients for all three forms are significant. Mean scores and tables of content analysis are provided as well.

**Tests of Articulation.** Articulation tests, such as those described below, measure only a fairly limited number of dimensions no matter how complex they may seem. These dimensions are place and manner of articulation, presence of voicing, elicited production or imitation, and phonemic context.

Which articulators, or speech organs, are involved in the production of the phoneme? The answer to such a question reveals the place of articulation. The articulators are usually assumed to be the lips, teeth, alveolar ridge (the area behind the upper teeth), palate, and tongue. When two of the articulators are brought together in the production of a phoneme, the place of contact between them is called the place of articulation. For example, /p/ is a bilabial phoneme, because it is produced by bringing the two lips together; /k/ is a lingua-palatal phoneme, because its production requires the tongue and palate to come into contact.

The manner of articulation refers to how the phoneme is produced. It may be with a puff of air, such as /p/ and /b/; with friction, as in /f/; or with hissing, as in /s/. As the reader can deduce, all of these sounds are produced with varying degrees of closure between articulators. The classes of closure are often categorized as stops (or plosives), fricatives, nasals, affricates, glides, and laterals.

Voicing is a very simple dimension of articulation denoting merely whether the phoneme is produced with or without vocal tone. All vowels are produced with voice, but the voicing feature is used as a description of consonants, because many of them are distinguished from one another only by the voicing feature, such as /p/ and /b/, /t/ and /d/, and /s/ and /z/.

A number of articulation tests allow for the assessment of sounds that are produced either spontaneously or only in imitation of the test administrator's production of the sound. Even if the test does not allow for imitation, most clinicians will use it.

Only a few commercial tests of articulation include techniques for distinctive feature analysis of phonemic errors. Such an analysis is a procedure for contrasting the features (manner and place of articulation and voicing) that may be represented in a child's articulation errors. For example, a feature analysis of a given child's articulation test profile could indicate that the child's errors are the result of the lack of a particular feature, such as the absence of the labio-dental feature in place of articulation.

At least two, and perhaps more, of the commercially available tests of articulation feature the assessment of phonemes within a variety of phonemic contexts. For example, in English the phoneme /r/ is never followed by the phoneme /s/ in single words; however, in contextual speech the combination may occur quite frequently as in the production of such word combinations as *barstool.* Testing phonemes in context often reveals contexts in which a defective phoneme is produced correctly, and that context can form a point of origin for therapy.

*Templin-Darley Test of Articulation.* The oldest test of articulation that is still used widely is probably the *Templin-Darley Diagnostic Test of Articulation* (Templin & Darley, 1969), which is based on the Templin (1957) normative data. It is a 141 item, single word test that is designed to elicit all phonemes in all positions (initial, medial, and final) and in common blends. As with almost all articulation tests, it is a picture presentation test, although for some older persons there are sentences that can be used. The score obtained by the child is the number of items produced correctly, and the score can be evaluated by comparing it with means and standard deviations that are given for each one-half year level from ages 3 to 5 years and at one year intervals from 5 to 8 years. The variables of sex and socioeconomic status are also considered in the norms. There is probably little value to the reliability and validity coefficients that are presented in the manual, because, in the last analysis, articulation tests are used diagnostically rather than formally by speech pathologists who have determined the presence of an articulation disorder prior to administering a lengthy diagnostic instrument. The data obtained from the test are used for therapeutic rather than identification purposes.

*A Deep Test of Articulation.* Another older and less frequently used test of articulation is McDonald's (1964) *A Deep Test of Articulation,* in which pairs of pictures or written sentences are presented to elicit the production of a phoneme in many different phonetic contexts. Using a screening test of any kind, the speech pathologist first determines the error sounds and then employs the appropriate combination of pictures or sentences to elicit the phoneme in about 30 different contexts in which the test phonemes comes after the context sound. For example, if the child manifests a defective /s/, the picture card *house* from the first pack of cards in the test is presented in combination with all of the picture cards from the second pack, each depicting a word that begins with a different sound. The child is instructed to say the unusual two-syllable words that are formed from pairing the two pictures, such as *housetie* or *housecow*. McDonald indicates that if the sound is produced correctly in 75% of the contexts, therapy is probably not necessary. Moreover, if therapy is necessary, it would probably be best to begin with those combinations in which the child produces the phoneme correctly.

*Goldman-Fristoe Test of Articulation.* The *Goldman-Fristoe Test of Articulation* (Goldman & Fristoe, 1969) samples both spontaneous and imitative phonemic production and includes both single word and conversational speech production. In addition, phonemes are assessed in the initial, medial, and final positions as appropriate. The test manual provides test-retest and interrater reliability percentages ranging from 71 to 100%. Percentile rank norms are given for males and females aged 6–0 to 16+ years on spontaneous production of words and on elicited production of syllables.

*Fisher-Logemann Test of Articulation Competence.* A test designed to assist in the assessment of distinctive features is the *Fisher-Logemann Test of Articulation Competence* (Fisher & Logemann, 1971). Three parameters were chosen for the analysis of the distinctive features of consonants and four parameters for the analysis of vowels. Voicing, place of articulation, and manner of articulation are analyzed in consonants; height of tongue, place of articulation, degree of tension, and lip rounding are evaluated in vowel production. The system of distinctive feature analysis presented by Jakobson, Fant, and Halle (1963) is not used by the authors, because they felt that it was much too complex for the routine articulation testing that is done by most school speech pathologists. Instead, the authors adapted the Jakobson approach and designed a much more simplified analysis.

The test consists of 109 pictures on 39 cards plus 15 sentences for children or adults who read. Consonants are tested in prevocalic position (before a vowel in a syllable), postvocalic position (after a vowel), and intervocalic position (between two vowels). The twelve vowels are tested in either single syllable words or in words with the test vowel receiving primary stress. In addition, 23 blends and four diphthongs are tested. As with most articulation tests, the test procedures and test data are similar to the Templin-Darley. One advantage to the test is that the test record blank is arranged to facilitate the analysis of distinctive features, thereby assisting the examiner in the interpretation of test results. One disadvantage of the test is that it may require a much higher degree of proficiency in phonetic transcription than many school speech pathologists possess.

*Test of Articulation Performance.* One of the most recently published articulation tests is the *Test of Articulation Performance* (Bryant & Bryant, 1983), which has both a standardized screening form (TAP–S) and an inventory for feature analysis (TAP–D). The diagnostic inventory is the most comprehensive of articulation tests in that it measures six different parameters of speech production: phonemes in isolated words, distinctive features, articulation of adjacent phonemes, phonemes in continuous speech, phonemic modeling, and the speaker's attitude toward his or her speech. The TAP–D incorporates elements of all of the tests previously discussed as well as adding the factor of attitude. Reliability coefficients for the TAP–S, ranging from .88 to .96, are given for internal consistency and test-retest reliability; interrater reliability is estimated at 95%. All components of the TAP–S were examined with regard to content, criterion related, and construct validity, as appropriate, and were determined to have significantly high validity coefficients. A readily apparent advantage of the TAP–D and the TAP–S is their comprehensiveness. The examiner is able to assess a variety of articulatory dimensions using a single instrument.

## Tests of Syntax and Semantics

In this section six standardized tests of language performance are discussed briefly. As opposed to the instruments discussed above, which were limited to the measurement of only a single language ability, these tests are generally much more comprehensive. For the most part they assess syntax and semantics in both comprehension and production modes; some measure other attributes as well. The selection of the tests for review was arbitrary, the major selection criterion was that they deal with language in a linguistic paradigm rather than in a psychological or even psycholinguistic model. For this reason one of the best known tests, the *Illinois Test of Psycholinguistic Abilities* (Kirk, McCarthy, & Kirk, 1968) was not chosen for inclusion, because it contains many visual and memory elements that are difficult to reference in a linguistic model.

All of the tests reviewed here have advantages and disadvantages. The primary advantage to all of them is that they are, for the most part, well-standardized. This gives the examiner a reliable reference point for identifying children who have language delays or disorders severe enough to warrant therapeutic intervention. The disadvantage of these tests and of all others like them is that they contain too few items to represent the domains measured and, therefore, cannot be used to inventory children's special needs. These tests may provide baseline information about the child's linguistic performance, but they do not thoroughly explore the deficits that the child may be manifesting. Such an investigation requires the use of other assessment techniques. However, the information obtained from the tests reviewed here is valuable when applied appropriately and should not be underrated.

Six tests are discussed in this section, but the reader is not to assume that these six are recommended over and above any other well-standardized measures. As stated before, they were selected because they are prototypes of standardized language tests and because they are commonly used by practitioners in the field. Table 5.1 presents a more comprehensive listing of various types of oral language measures for the reader who would like to make some comparisons among instruments.

*Test for Auditory Comprehension of Language.* The TACL (Carrow, 1973) is a very popular test that purports to measure a number of lexical and structural elements in both English and Spanish. The language categories measured by the TACL are (a) form classes and function words, (b) morphological constructions, (c) grammatical categories, and (d) syntactic structure. Each of these categories may contain four to seven subcategories, and each subcategory may be assessed with only 1 to 18 items, the average being 4.21 items per subcategory. For subcategories like nouns that have 12 items, adjectives with 18 items, and verbs with 8 items, there may be enough test items to warrant making conclusions regarding the child's performance in these areas. However, when a subcategory like interrogatives is tested with only 3 items, conclusions cannot be made regarding the child's knowledge in that area. The test has value because it is one of the few standardized linguistic measures that can be used with Spanish-speaking children. Means and standard deviations are given for four test components: lexical, morphological, grammatical, and syntactical subtests and for the total for children at the kindergarten and first grade levels. Reliability coefficients indicate that the total score and all subtest scores except the syntactic are adequate.

*Test of Adolescent Language.* The TOAL (Hammill, Brown, Larsen, & Wiederholt, 1987) is the only standardized, nationally normed test of language for students aged 11–1 to 18–11 years. It is a comprehensive test composed of eight subtests that measure the expressive and receptive components of reading and writing and the lexical and grammatic aspects of listening and speaking. In addition to providing subtest scores, the instrument allows the examiner to calculate a number of composite scores, such as those for spoken language, written language, receptive language, expressive language, vocabulary, grammar, and a number of others. Coefficients for internal, test-retest, and interrater reliability are all high, and the test is a valuable addition to the examiner's repertoire of language tests.

*Clinical Evaluation of Language Functions.* The CELF (Semel & Wiig, 1980) is composed of eleven subtests that measure certain aspects of language in the areas of semantics (word meanings), syntax (sentence structure), and memory (recall and retrieval). In addition, two subtests are devoted to the assessment of phonology (articulation and discrimination of speech sounds). The CELF Screening Test was standardized on a stratified sample of 1,405

**TABLE 5.1. Tests of Oral Language**

| Test | Purpose | | Elements | | |
|---|---|---|---|---|---|
| | Identification | Instruction | Phonology | Syntax | Semantics |
| *Auditory Discrimination Test* (Wepman, 1958) | X | | X | | |
| *Assessment of Children's Language Comprehension* (Foster, Giddan, & Stark, 1972) | X | X | | X | X |
| *Basic Concept Inventory* (Englemann, 1967) | X | | | | X |
| *Birth to Three Developmental Scale* (Bangs & Dodson, 1979) | X | X | | X | X |
| *Carrow Elicited Language Inventory* (Carrow, 1974) | X | X | | X | X |
| *Clinical Evaluation of Language Functions* (Semel & Wiig, 1980) | X | | | X | X |
| *Denver Developmental Screening Test* (Frankenburg, Dodds, Fandal, Kazuk, & Cohrs, 1975) | X | | | X | X |
| *Developmental Activities Screening Inventory* (Fewell & Langley, 1984) | X | | | X | X |
| *Developmental Sentence Analysis* (Lee, 1974) | X | X | | X | |
| *Fisher-Logemann Test of Articulation Competence* (Fisher & Logemann, 1971) | X | X | X | | |

**TABLE 5.1.** continued

| | | | | | |
|---|---|---|---|---|---|
| *Goldman-Fristoe Test of Articulation* (Goldman & Fristoe, 1969) | X | X | X | | |
| *Illinois Test of Psycholinguistic Abilities* (Kirk, McCarthy, & Kirk, 1968) | X | | | X | X |
| *Language-Related Tests of Speech-Sound Discrimination* (Bryen, 1974) | X | | X | | |
| *Linguistic Analysis of Speech Samples* (Angler, Hannah, & Longhurst, 1973) | X | X | | X | X |
| *Miller-Yoder Test of Grammatical Comprehension* (Miller & Yoder, 1972) | X | X | | X | |
| *Minnesota Child Development Inventory* (Ireton & Thwing, 1972) | X | | | X | X |
| *Northwestern Syntax Screening Test* (Lee, 1969) | X | | | X | |
| *Peabody Picture Vocabulary Test* (Dunn, 1981) | X | | | | X |
| *Screening Test of Spanish Grammar* (Toronto, 1973) | X | | | X | |
| *Templin-Darley Tests of Articulation* (Templin & Darley, 1969) | X | X | X | | |
| *Test for Auditory Comprehension of Language* (Carrow, 1973) | X | | | X | X |
| *Test of Adolescent Language* (Hammill, Brown, Larsen, & Wiederholt, 1987) | X | | | X | X |

**TABLE 5.1.** continued

| | | | | | |
|---|---|---|---|---|---|
| *Test of Articulation Performance* (Bryant & Bryant, 1983) | X | X | X | | |
| *Test of Early Language Development* (Hresko, Reid, & Hammill, 1981) | X | | | X | X |
| *Test of Language Development–Intermediate* (Hammill & Newcomer, 1982) | X | | X | X | X |
| *Test of Language Development–Primary* (Newcomer & Hammill, 1982) | X | | X | X | X |
| *Utah Test of Language Development* (Mecham, Jex, & Jones, 1973) | X | | | | X |
| *Verbal Language Development Scale* (Mecham, 1958) | X | | | | X |
| *Vocabulary Comprehension Scale* (Bangs, 1977) | X | | | | X |

Adapted from *Learning Disabilities: Basic Concepts, Assessment Practices, and Instructional Strategies* (pp. 56–57) by P. Myers and D. Hammill, 1982, Austin, TX: PRO-ED. Reprinted by permission.

children in grades K–12; however, the Diagnostic Battery was standardized on only 159 of the students who took the Screening Test. It would appear that the reliability coefficients, which are all within acceptable limits, should be viewed with some reservations due to the small size of the sample used. The validity coefficients are also open to the same criticism.

The CELF has some interesting variations, particularly those that allow for evaluation of grammaticality and complexity and the subtests that allow for probes of incorrect responses. The test manual also contains a number of appendixes, some of which are particularly useful, such as the description of dialectical variations in morphology and syntax and the overview of informal extension testing formats at the syntactic level.

*Test of Early Language Development.* The TELD (Hresko, Reid, & Hammill, 1981) measures spoken language in the expressive and receptive modes for the dimensions of content and form. Content is defined as a semantic dimension and is related to the expression or reception of word meaning, conceptual categories, and interpretation of meaning within varying contexts. The dimension of form refers to syntax, morphology, and phonology. The TELD was standardized on 1,184 children between the ages of 3–0 and 7–11 years. Reliability coefficients for internal and test-retest reliability are within acceptable limits. Content, criterion related, and construct validity were examined, and the authors state that the validity of the test is well supported.

*Clark-Madison Test of Oral Language.* The Clark-Madison (Clark & Madison, 1981) is designed for young children ages 4–0 and 8–11 years and is one of the most widely used tests of spoken language in early childhood education programs. It was developed to assess young children's expressive abilities in various grammatical and syntactic components of language as well as target modifiers, determiners, prepositions, verbs, pronouns, and inflections. It uses a unique nominative elicitation technique in its administration. The authors have reviewed much of the research related to the relationship between spontaneous language sampling and structured elicitation. They found that the nominative elicitation technique as used in the Clark-Madison test results in children producing 52% of the target structures that were not produced when spontaneous speech samples were taken.

To understand the item administration technique better, a couple of examples are given. The child is shown a picture of a boy carrying a large box and two boys carrying some small boxes between them. The examiner points to the first picture and says, "Listen. His box is big." The examiner then points to the second picture and says, "Tell me about them." The correct response is, "Their boxes are small," in which the target item is *their* or *theirs*. As one might expect, demonstration items are scattered throughout the test because, as the authors concede, the administration technique places large demands on the child's memory capacity. The authors give some examples of how poor memory may affect the child's responses and suggest that if a memory deficit is thought to be interfering with the administration of the test, some other measurement device should be used.

The authors recognize that the standardization sample of 144 children is of minimal size, and they report that extensive standardization and normative data analysis is underway. The reliability and validity coefficients as reported in the 1981 test manual are within acceptable limits but should be viewed with reservation because of the small sample size.

*Test of Language Development–Primary* and *Test of Language Development–Intermediate.* The TOLD–P (Newcomer & Hammill, 1982) and the TOLD–I (Hammill & Newcomer, 1982) are very widely used measures of oral language that have been carefully standardized and normed. The tests employ a two-dimensional model of language function to measure the receptive and expressive modes of phonology, syntax, and semantics. The TOLD tests have been used as the criteria in many studies examining the criterion related validity of other tests because of their excellent construction and statistical characteristics.

Reliability coefficients for internal and test-retest reliability are quite high, as are the validity coefficients. The TOLD was meticulously standardized, and a great deal of statistical information is available in the test manuals.

## A Statement on the Results of Standardized Testing

Therapists, diagnosticians, and other appraisal personnel know that it is often difficult to determine whether a child has a language disorder. The great advantage to standardized tests, for the experienced professional as well as for the novice, is that they are often excellent tools for identifying broad areas of language disability. When a test is well standardized and well normed, it can be used to answer the primary diagnostic question: Does the child have a problem? At the same time, the examiner must remember that in the moderately or severely delayed youngster, the characteristics of mental retardation, cultural deprivation, emotional disturbance, and language disorder can be misinterpreted. The examiner cannot always be sure what is the origin of the language deficiency. The child has a problem to be sure, but what is the nature of that problem? What is the most appropriate intervention? What are the skills to be taught? What are the reasonable expectations for progress? These are not questions answered by the kinds of standardized tests discussed above. To be fair, the test authors do not usually indicate that their tests supply such answers. More generally, authors caution the examiner against making such diagnostic or instructional inferences. Answers to many of the diagnostic questions surrounding an oral language disorder can be discovered only through informal criterion referenced assessment, involving observation and elicitation of speech samples in a variety of contexts, and diagnostic teaching. The remaining sections of this chapter deal with the analysis of language or speech samples and other testing techniques.

## ANALYSIS OF LANGUAGE SAMPLES

The analysis of spontaneous speech samples was first advocated as an assessment tool by McCarthy (1930), who used the child's output as a basis for calculating the mean length of response and for analyzing structural complexity and vocabulary. Since that time many authors have used language samples in both structured and unstructured analyses of children's linguistic behavior. The analysis of language samples taken over a period of time in varying situations exemplifies the holistic or molar approach to assessment, although obviously, even the analysis of a language sample can be done in a highly specific, molecular fashion. It is important to remember that any language assessment should provide the examiner with the maximum amount of information about the total language functioning of the child and with data related to all aspects of the child's behavior as he or she interacts verbally and nonverbally with the environment.

The discussion of language samples is divided into four sections: (a) collecting and recording the language sample; (b) information on the appropriate size of the sample; (c) analysis of linguistic elements; and (d) interpretation of the mean length of utterance (MLU).

### Collecting and Recording the Language Sample

Much of the information in this section is adapted from Miller (1981), who gives a detailed explanation of the use of language samples in assessment. Miller acknowledges that the most difficult part of collecting a free-speech sample, particularly with very young or developmentally delayed children, is initiating the therapist-child interaction and convincing the child that he or she wants to talk to the therapist. Some of the strategies advocated are as follows:

1. Do not say anything to the child after the first friendly greeting for the first five minutes of the interaction.

2. Engage in parallel play with the child for the first few minutes but do very little talking. It is suggested that this is a very effective technique with children who are functioning at a cognitive level below 30 months.

3. Engage in interactive play with the child but still do little talking. This works best with children at the 3 to 5 year cognitive level.

4. Finally, engage in interactive play without an introduction. Simply begin playing with the child and then invite discussion after the activity is finished.

Usually, one of these strategies will be effective in initiating the child's speech production; if not, the clinician may need to enlist the participation of the child's mother, a sibling, or another child. Children must feel comfortable, and it is important not to pressure them. With many recalcitrant children, the pressure applied on them to make them talk will result in even greater resistance, and the entire session may have to be abandoned.

Language samples can be collected in almost any setting in which the child is comfortable and, for very young children, should probably be collected in more than one setting to obtain a representative sample. It appears that older children (at least 3 to 4 years old) produce quite representative samples in the clinical setting. The clinician should keep in mind that the sample should be representative of the child's linguistic development and that certain settings tend to evoke only limited types of language production. For example, a sample taken in a classroom will often reflect classroom language behavior: questions during working time, declaratives during "show and tell."

The materials used during the collection of a language sample should be varied, and, if possible, some toys new to the child should be provided. Certain types of games are not productive because they tend to evoke rote types of utterances. For example, playing with Old Maid cards will usually result in very limited, routine productions; playing games will often evoke nothing more than, "It's your turn," or counting; and picture books can lead to routines such as "Once upon a time, there were three little pigs."

The language sample can be recorded in several manners: shorthand or speedwriting, audiotape recordings, or videotape recordings. The first, manual transcription, is not recommended unless recording equipment is unavailable or impractical to use. It is very difficult to write down everything that children say unless their verbal output is quite small. Probably the most effective method is using the audiotape recorder. The microphone may inhibit children initially, although not nearly as much as will a videotape recorder. Some time should be spent showing the equipment to the children and letting them get used to it. It is best to use multidirectional microphones placed about one to two feet from the child instead of lavalior or tie-tack microphones, which are restrictive to movement and are distracting.

## Size of Language Sample

The examiner may take two approaches to the question of language sample size: either specify the number of utterances at 50, 100, or 200 or specify the amount of time that will be devoted to taking a sample. Miller (1981) recommends the latter approach because he feels it has greater flexibility. Using 30 minutes as the time for interaction, about 100 to 200 utterances can be produced by children functioning at 24 months of age and up. Children functioning below that level will produce fewer than 100 utterances, with children between 18 and 24 months producing about 30 to 60 utterances. Children who are functioning between 12 and 18 months will produce very few utterances, and samples should be supplemented either by the parents at home or by the clinician in ongoing sessions.

Even though a very good microphone may be used for recording every utterance the child produces and though transcription may be highly accurate, it is still important for the clinician to make contextual notes during the session. Bloom (1970) underlines the necessity for keeping a record of the child's activities while he or she is producing the utterances. Bloom's classic example of the utterance, "Mommy sock," could not have been interpreted without knowing that the child produced the utterance while holding the mother's sock, thus indicating a possessive relationship. If the child were holding his or her own sock, speaking with proper stress, and indicating *mother*, one could infer an agent-object request ("Mommy, put on my sock"). To further ensure that the context of the child's utterances is preserved, the transcription of the sample must include the examiner's utterances as well as the child's. Figure 5.1 shows the type of transcription format used by Miller (1981).

## Analysis of Linguistic Elements

A number of authors have suggested various methods of analyzing linguistic elements in a language sample. Table 5.2, taken from Miller (1981), details some of those procedures, the linguistic elements that have been quantified, the size of the language sample that is advised, and the age range for which the procedure may be used. Table 5.3 is a listing of measures that rely on a language sample as the primary source of data for assessment.

Of the measures detailed in Table 5.2, probably the most useful is the mean length of utterance (MLU), a time-honored method of analyzing children's free speech. Mean length of utterance, as a quantifiable indicator of children's linguistic capacity, is better understood if Brown's (1973) description of the stages of language development is considered.

**Counting Rules for the Mean Length of Utterance.** In calculating and interpreting the MLU, one uses the guidelines provided by Chapman

## FIGURE 5.1. Format for Transcription of Language Sample

Name of child: Mark
Clinic number: ________
Chronological age: 6–8
Date of evaluation: ________
Examiners: ________

Key:

| | | |
|---|---|---|
| C = Child | [ ] | Gloss or Contextual notes |
| E = Examiner | ( ) | Questionable Transcription |
| XXX = unintelligible | / / | Phonetic Transcription |
| . . . = pause | | |

Situation variables:
Time of day: 1:30 p.m.
Setting: Waisman Center (Rm. 145)
Materials used: Blocks, puzzle, PAT pictures, DLM pictures, puppet
Length of interaction: 18 minutes
Participants/Type of interactions: 1. Clinician-child
2. ________
3. ________
4. ________

Child MLU: 2.50
Number of utterances: 53
Number of intelligible utterances: 52
Sources of transcription: Audiotape

Adult MLU: ________
1. Mother ________
2. Clinician ________
3. ________

**FIGURE 5.1.** continued

| Pragmatics | | Speaker | Utterance Number | Dialogue | Morpheme Count | | Syntax | Semantics |
|---|---|---|---|---|---|---|---|---|
| Child | Adult | | | | Child | Adult | | |
| | | C | 1. Hey, that Cookie Monster stands. | | | | | |
| | | E | | 1. That stands? | | | | |
| | | | | 2. It sure does. | | | | |
| | | | | 3. Mark, do you know who this is? | | | | |
| | | C | 2. Oscar. | | | | | |
| | | E | | 4. Is that Oscar? | | | | |
| | | | | 5. Or is that the Cookie Monster? | | | | |
| | | C | 3. Oscar. | | | | | |
| | | E | | 6. Oscar! | | | | |
| | | C | 4. Cookie Monster in there. [box] | | | | | |
| | | E | | 7. The Cookie Monster's in there? | | | | |
| | | | | 8. I thought this was the Cookie Monster? | | | | |
| | | C | [shakes head] | | | | | |

From *Assessing Language Production in Children: Experimental Procedures* (p. 15) by J. Miller, 1981, Austin, TX: PRO-ED.

TABLE 5.2. General Analysis Procedures for Quantifying Transcripts of Free-Speech Samples

| Content | Measure | Sample size advised | Range of use | Reference |
|---|---|---|---|---|
| Syntax | Mean Length of Utterance in Morphemes (MLU) | 50 utterances or more | 1.5–5 years | Brown, 1973; this volume |
| | Mean Length of Utterance in Words (MLR) | 50 utterances | 1.5–8 years | Templin, 1957 |
| | Mean Length of T-unit or Communication Unit (MLTR) | 30 T-units | 5–18 years | Loban, 1976 |
| | Frequency distribution—Number of utterances by length | 50 utterances[a] | 1.5–18 years | This volume |
| | Frequency distribution—Number of utterances by structural type | 50 utterances[a] | 1.5–18 years | This volume |
| | Developmental Sentence Score (DSS) | 50 utterances or more | 3–7 years | Lee, 1974 |
| | Length-Complexity Index (LCI) | 15–50 utterances | 4–8 years | Shriner, 1967, 1969; Miner, 1969; Barlow and Miner, 1969; Griffith and Miner, 1969 |
| Semantics | Type-Token Ratio–Vocabularity Diversity | 50 utterances or more | 3–8 years | Templin, 1957 |

**TABLE 5.2.** continued

| | | | | |
|---|---|---|---|---|
| Phonology | Percent intelligible, partially intelligible, and unintelligible utterances | 50 utterances[a] | 1–18 years | |
| Communicative interaction | Frequency distribution of number of utterances per speaking turn for each | | | |
| | speaker, Mom's MLU- | 50 utterances[a] | | |
| | Child's MLU ratio, number | 50 utterances[a] | 1–18 years | Retherford, Schwartz, and Chapman, in press |
| | of Mom's utterances to number of Child's | 50 utterances[a] | 1.5–5 years | |
| | utterances | 50 utterances[a] | 2–18 years | Retherford, Schwartz, and Chapman, in press |

[a]Number of utterances may vary for these analysis procedures. Fifty utterances is considered a minimum target providing enough data for interpretation. Note that as sample size increases, representativeness is likely to increase.

From *Assessing Language Production in Children: Experimental Procedures* (p. 23) by J. Miller, 1981, Austin, TX: PRO-ED. Reprinted by permission.

**TABLE 5.3. Measures of Spontaneous Language Analysis Procedures**

| Measure | Author |
|---|---|
| Mean length of utterance (MLU) | McCarthy (1970) |
| Length-complexity index | Miner (1969) |
| Developmental sentence types (DST) | Lee (1966) |
| Linguistic analysis of speech samples (LASS) | Engler, Hannah, & Lonehurst (1973) |
| Co-occurring and restricted structure procedure (CORS) | Muma (1973) |
| Developmental sentence scoring (DSS) | Lee (1974) |
| Tyack and Gottsleben's language analysis system | Tyack & Gottsleben (1974) |
| Grammatical analysis of language disability | Crystal, Fletcher, & Garman (1976) |
| Trantham and Pederson's modified DSS | Trantham & Pederson (1976) |
| Case relation analysis | Scroggs (1977) |
| Language sample analysis | Bloom & Lahey (1978) |
| Assigning structural stage (ASS) | Miller (1981) |

From "Assessment of Language Disorders: Linguistic and Cognitive Functions" by D. Geffner, 1981, *Topics in Language Disorders, I,* pp. 1–10. Reprinted by permission of Aspen Publishers.

(in Miller, 1981), who says that the first consecutive 50 intelligible morphemes in the sample are counted. The reader should recall that a morpheme is a minimal meaningful unit of language; for example, *dogs* consists of two morphemes, *dog* and the plural *-s.* The counting rules given below are adapted from Brown (1973) and Chapman.

1. *Repetitions.* If stuttering occurs it should be noted, but the word is counted only once. If a word is repeated for emphasis, it should be counted each time.
2. *Fillers.* Utterances such as *mm* or *uh* are not counted; actual words, even though used as fillers, such as *yeah* or *no,* are counted.

3. *Compound words, proper names, and reduplications.* Each is counted as a single word, even though it may consist of two utterances, such as *tick-tock, John Brown,* or *seesaw.*

4. *Irregular past tense.* Verbs in the irregular past tense, such as *did, went, saw,* and so on, are counted as single morphemes because there is no evidence that children view them as anything separate from the present tense.

5. *Diminutives.* All count as one word because diminutives are standard forms for children.

6. *Auxiliaries and concatenations.* All are counted as separate, single words. Concatenations, such as *gonna, hafta,* and so on, are standard forms for children and are only representations for *going to, have to,* and so on. All inflections, such as regular past *-ed,* progressive *-ing,* possessive *-e,* plural *-s,* and third person singular *-s,* are counted as separate morphemes.

**Checking the Validity of the Mean Length of Utterance.** Transcripts of samples should be checked to investigate their representativeness of the MLU. Several characteristics can affect the MLU by either inflating or deflating it. If more than 20% of the child's utterances are imitations of the previous speaker, the MLU may be spuriously high. To check this, one may calculate separate MLUs for the imitations and for the spontaneous utterances.

If self-repetitions occur frequently in the sample, the MLU may be higher than warranted. Brown (1973) included these utterances, but Bloom (1973) excluded them. One way to check the validity of the MLU is to calculate it with and without the self-repetitions similar to the method suggested for checking on imitations. A high proportion of questions-answers in the sample will tend to reduce spontaneous speech and may deflate the child's MLU. In collecting the sample, try to keep the questioning technique at a minimum, or the sample may consist of a great many *Yes, No,* and *Here* responses.

Some children's language samples may be marked by a high proportion of what are termed *routines* (i.e., nursery rhymes, commercial jingles, alphabets, counting, etc.). The MLU may be upwardly biased by the inclusion of these utterances. Again, the procedure recommended by Brown is to calculate the MLU with and without the routines. It is not uncommon for language samples reflecting MLUs of 4.0 to 5.0 or higher to contain frequent instances of sentence conjunction. Older children commonly use run-on sentences, continually beginning a new sentence with "And then." Chapman (in Miller, 1981) recommends that the MLU not be computed for such children but that other utterance measures be used that are better designed to assess the increasing grammatical sophistication of the child. One of the measures that might be used is the T-unit or communication unit count described by

Loban (1976), which treats each clause headed by *and* as a single unit of communication.

To compute the MLU, first count the total number of morphemes produced and then divide by the total number of utterances counted, as shown in the formula below:

$$\text{MLU} = \frac{\text{Number of Morphemes}}{\text{Number of Utterances}} \quad \text{or} \quad \text{MLU} = \frac{\text{M}}{\text{U}}$$

Recall that an utterance is similar to a sentence but is not the same as what we consider an adult sentence. Utterances will have to be marked off by using the criterion of terminal intonation contour—falling intonation for declarative utterance, rising for interrogative.

## Interpretation of the Mean Length of Utterance

The MLU is a valuable index only if it represents the child's normal discourse. Some suggestions were given above as to ways that representativeness can be investigated. Some other factors that can affect the MLU are the child's familiarity with the examiner, the setting itself, the topic of discourse, the child's present health and mood, and so on. The MLU is a general indicator of structural language development and can be reliably interpreted only when it falls between 1.01 and 4.49 morphemes. Two methods of interpretation of the MLU are structural stages and distributional analysis.

**Stages of Structural Development.** The MLU is interpreted in terms of Brown's stages I through V. Each stage, as discussed in Chapter 4, is associated with distinct developmental achievements and defines the predictable structures in the child's expressive language. An MLU of 2.80 places the child at Stage III, while an MLU of 4.30 reflects Stage V development. As may be seen in Table 4.8, the former MLU gives a child a predicted chronological age of 33.2 months and the latter an age of 45.0 months. By the same token, the examiner is able to predict the MLU and MLU ranges within one standard deviation for children 18 to 60 months of age by using Miller's (1981) data shown in Table 5.4. Miller notes that the data shown in tables 4.8 and 5.4 should not be considered exhaustively normative, because the sample upon which they are based was a relatively small sample of middle-class children from Madison, Wisconsin. Although the data may not be generalized to all populations of young children, they do give the examiner a starting point for estimating MLU or predicting chronological age.

**Distributional Analysis.** Another way of analyzing the MLU and the language sample as a whole is to reorganize the transcript of the sample

**TABLE 5.4. Predicted MLUs and MLU Ranges Within One Standard Deviation of Predicted Mean for Each Age Group**

| Age ±1 Month | Predicted MLU[a] | Predicted SD[b] | Predicted MLU ±1 SD (middle 68%) |
|---|---|---|---|
| 18 | 1.31 | 0.325 | 0.99–1.64 |
| 21 | 1.62 | 0.386 | 1.23–2.01 |
| 24 | 1.92 | 0.448 | 1.47–2.37 |
| 30 | 2.54 | 0.571 | 1.97–3.11 |
| 33 | 2.85 | 0.633 | 2.22–3.48 |
| 36 | 3.16 | 0.694 | 2.47–3.85 |
| 39 | 3.47 | 0.756 | 2.71–4.23 |
| 42 | 3.78 | 0.817 | 2.96–4.60 |
| 45 | 4.09 | 0.879 | 3.21–4.97 |
| 48 | 4.40 | 0.940 | 3.46–5.34 |
| 51 | 4.71 | 1.002 | 3.71–5.71 |
| 54 | 5.02 | 1.064 | 3.96–6.08 |
| 57 | 5.32 | 1.125 | 4.20–6.45 |
| 60 | 5.63 | 1.187 | 4.44–6.82 |

[a]MLU is predicted from the equation MLU = −0.548 + 0.103 (age).
[a]SD is predicted from the equation $SD_{MLU}$ = −0.0446 + 0.0205 (age).

From *Assessing Language Production in Children: Experimental Procedures* (p. 27) by J. Miller, 1981, Austin, TX: PRO-ED.

by specific utterance characteristics. Some of the segments that Chapman (in Miller, 1981) recommends are (a) sentence length, (b) syntactic structures, and (c) number of utterances per speaking turn. If one reorganizes the transcript by sentence length, the MLU will be clarified by quantifying the number of utterances of each length that were produced. There are variations around the mean to be expected, but a number of spuriously long sentences may seriously inflate the MLU, and the examiner should consider such MLUs invalid.

A distributional analysis by syntactic structures provides the examiner with data regarding the structural variety in the child's language production. One favored technique is known as Assigning Structural State (ASS), but any type of sample segmentation that reveals the variety and number of syntactic structures used by the child would be acceptable. Some children may generate enough words and utterances to obtain a fairly high MLU, but an analysis of their syntactic structures may reveal a significant degree of poverty in the variety of structures produced.

The third distributional analysis that the examiner could use requires segmenting the language sample into the number of utterances produced by the child in each of his or her turns to speak. This involves analysis on a more pragmatic level of language. The number of the utterances produced by both the child and the examiner is segmented; the relationship between the two reflects the distribution of talking for each and the child's turn-taking ability in discourse. It may also indicate how much the examiner (or other adult) allowed the child to talk.

Although the language sample can be analyzed in a number of ways not described here (see Miller, 1981), the procedures given above are the usual techniques discussed by most authors for analyzing free-speech samples of children.

## USING INFORMAL ASSESSMENT PROCEDURES

Standardized or nonstandardized (informal) approaches to language assessment are chosen according to the reason for assessment. The first question to be asked is why a child is being evaluated. Is information needed to decide whether the child's language is deviant? If so, quantitative, normed, standardized approaches are valuable in supplying the answer. If, however, the question is related to the direction that intervention should take, the informal approaches are beneficial in generating courses of therapy. The standardized measures, such as those discussed in the previous section, can resolve the question of deviance through comparison with norms but can provide little information about the parameters of the problem or the type of therapy needed. Similarly, because of the lack of normative data, informal tasks give little information regarding the question of deviance.

Some of the informal assessment procedures discussed in this section yield a type of age-related information, but the strength of the procedures lies in their flexibility and in their usefulness for designing an intervention program. The clinician must decide what the assessment questions are and then use the best measures to resolve those questions.

In this section, informal assessment procedures are described for the following areas of the oral language evaluation: assessment of language comprehension, assessment of language production, and assessment of pragmatics. All of the procedures found in this section are informal because they lack both standardization of administration and normative data. The examiner should feel free to adapt, extend, or in any other way modify the assessment procedures, suggested materials, and/or number of items.

## Assessment of Language Comprehension

Language comprehension is often assessed before language production because of the almost universally accepted dictum that reception precedes expression. Therefore, most clinicians feel that the investigation of the child's receptive or comprehension abilities gives significant clues as to what areas of production can and should be explored.

If the child is not "hard to assess," it is common practice to administer standardized tests, such as those described in a previous section. In this section, we will discuss other procedures that can be followed to assess in depth the child's speech sound discrimination, understanding of vocabulary, and comprehension of syntactic/semantic elements.

**Speech Sound Discrimination.** According to Aungst and Frick (1964), at least four types of auditory discrimination tasks are important for speech production: (a) matching two externally produced sounds, (b) matching an external sound to one produced by the child, (c) matching an external speech sound to an internal criterion, and (d) matching an internally produced sound with an internal criterion. The tasks are arranged in order of increasing difficulty. The first type of discrimination is probably the easiest, and often children with severe articulatory deficiencies can perform well on such a task. Matching two externally produced sounds is the paradigm followed by Wepman (1958) in the *Auditory Discrimination Test* and by most other authors of speech sound discrimination tests.

The second task that the clinician may ask the child to perform is matching an external speech sound to a sound produced by the child. The clinician produces the speech sound, and the child imitates it. Then the child is asked to determine whether the two sounds are the same or different. The sounds used should be those that the child is misarticulating. If the child is unable to tell whether his or her imitation matches the sound produced by the clinician, it will be difficult for correction to take place through imitation.

The next task is for the child to determine whether two sounds produced in syllables and words are correct or incorrect. To monitor and evaluate the clinician's speech sound production, the child must have an internal auditory image of the correct production to compare with what is heard. For some children, this task may be fairly easy, because it does not require that they monitor their own speech.

In the last type of discrimination task, the child produces the targeted sound and then judges whether the production was accurate. Successful performance on this task indicates that the child is able to monitor his or her own speech; failure would suggest that the child is unable to listen to and evaluate his or her speech production.

**Vocabulary.** Formal tests of vocabulary comprehension, such as those mentioned previously, reveal whether the child's understanding of single words is adequate for his or her age. If the test results indicate that the child's understanding of words is significantly impaired, the clinician should endeavor to discover whether this is a generalized deficit or whether the child's lack of comprehension is restricted to certain classes or categories of words. The classes of words should be both linguistic and cognitive. The following abbreviated chart (Table 5.5) contains a number of such classes of words for which the clinician can devise a picture test. For older children, the number of classes could be extended, and the accompanying words could be more difficult.

The pictures depicting the various words should be presented in the same fashion as the picture plates for the *Peabody Picture Vocabulary Test* (Dunn, 1981). At least four pictures should be presented to the child in random order. The child is asked to point to the picture named, and the clinician determines whether the child is responding incorrectly to certain classes of words or to a large number of unspecified words.

If possible, the clinician should also compare the child's vocabulary comprehension with his or her vocabulary production as expressed in ongoing language samples. In the usual course of language development, children's comprehension vocabularies far outstrip their expressive vocabularies in both numbers of words and complexity. If this is not the case, the clinician must examine or arrange for the evaluation of the child's intellectual and emotional status. That is not to say that the child may not have a language disorder, but it is an indicator that the child might be mentally retarded or emotionally disturbed rather than, or in addition to, being language disordered. The clinician must also consider the possibility of a hearing loss, but it should go without saying that any child being referred for oral language assessment should first be given a thorough audiological examination.

**Syntax/Semantics.** No attempt will be made to separate the components of syntax and semantics in the assessment of oral language comprehension; the two are inextricably interwoven. As only one example of this correlation between the two, consider the plural noun and its phonological, syntactic, and semantic properties. An analysis of the plurality of the words *cat* and *dog* follows:

1. *Phonological elements:* The plural of *cat* is formed by adding the phoneme /s/, while the plural of *dog* requires the addition of the phoneme /z/.

2. *Syntactic elements:* The plurals of both *cat* and *dog* are characterized by the addition of only the appropriate morpheme, not specifying which phoneme, and are shown schematically by *cat* + */-s/* or *dog* + */-s/*.

3. *Semantic elements:* No distinction is made between the plural of *cat* and *dog*. The criterion is that the child have the concept of plurality or "more than one." As the reader can easily see, asking the child to identify a plural requires at least syntactic and semantic knowledge from the child; asking him or her to produce a plural also requires phonological knowledge.

Bellugi-Klima (1971) suggests a variety of ways in which the clinician can assess syntactic structures that are known to children. The procedures

**TABLE 5.5. A List of Example Classes and Words to be Used in Assessing Vocabulary Comprehension**

| CLASSES | | | |
|---|---|---|---|
| **Cognitive[1]** | **Words[2]** | **Linguistic[3]** | **Words[2]** |
| Animals | Cat<br>Dog<br>Rabbit | Nouns | Box<br>Car<br>Train |
| Furniture | Bed<br>Chair<br>Sofa | Action Verbs | Running<br>Catch<br>Shove |
| Toys | Doll<br>Teddy Bear<br>Choo-choo | Pronouns | She<br>It<br>Our |
| People | Man<br>Woman<br>Lady | Prepositions | On<br>Beneath<br>Over |
| Family | Mother<br>Father<br>Sister | Adjectives | Pretty<br>Bad<br>Big |
| Occupations | Teacher<br>Policeman<br>Farmer | Adverbs | Quietly<br>Quickly<br>Very |
| Geographical Features | Hill<br>Mountain<br>Valley | | |

[1]Can be extended upwards developmentally through adding more abstract classes
[2]Can be extended by using more difficult vocabulary
[3]Can be extended by adding more complex linguistic classes

require that situational clues be eliminated from the presentation of the tasks, that the child know the vocabulary being presented, that the objects used in assessment be familiar to the child, and that the construction of the task require an understanding of the syntax of the sentences presented rather than some other feature. Bellugi-Klima's general approach entails providing the child with a number of familiar objects, producing a sentence, and asking the child to act out the meaning of the sentence. As an example, the passive construction can be tested by giving the child a boy and a girl doll, presenting two sentences that differ only in the syntax, and having the child demonstrate the meaning of the sentences (e.g., "The boy is pushed by the girl" and "The girl is pushed by the boy") by manipulating the dolls. It is possible to assess a number of syntactic structures in this fashion. The following tasks are some of those recommended by Bellugi-Klima.

*Active sentences.* In the majority of English sentences, the first noun is the subject (or actor), and the noun following the verb is the object or recipient of the action. The first question to be asked in the assessment of syntax is, "Given a verb, does the child know that the first noun is the actor and the second noun is the object?" Test as follows:

- Place a number of small objects before the child.
- Determine that the child knows what the objects are and knows the names of each.
- Determine that the child knows the meaning of the verbs that will be presented.
- Present two sentences that differ only in the subject-object relationship.
- Ask the child to demonstrate the meaning of the sentence by manipulating the objects.

*Examples:*

Show me: The boy feeds the girl.
Show me: The girl feeds the boy.

The general testing instructions will not be repeated for each of the syntactic structures that are discussed in this section, but the clinician should be sure to follow the procedures for all tasks.

*Singular/plural noun.* The inflection on the plural noun is one of the earliest inflections to appear in children's language development. In some cases the plural inflection on the noun is redundant, as there are other clues in the sentences. For example, the use of a plural copula *are*, plural demonstratives *these* and *those*, a plural such as *some*, and plural adjectives like *two* all signal plurality. Such words should be avoided in presenting assessment tasks; the sentences used should contain no other cues to plurality beyond the plural inflection on the noun.

*Examples:*

Give me the ball.
Give me the balls.

Give me the flower.
Give me the flowers.

Give me the cat.
Give me the cats.

*Possessive.* The possessive inflection of nouns occurs after the plural inflection, even though noun plus noun constructions (e.g., "Mommy dress") do appear fairly early in development. In assessing possessives, test the child's understanding of the fact that two nouns occur, the first being a modification of the second. In such cases, it is the second noun that is the head noun of the noun phrase. Instead of saying, "the girl's dress," one could paraphrase the sentence to say, "The dress that belongs to the girl." To assess the possessive, the clinician can set up minimal pairs as follows:

*Examples:*

Show me the girl's mommy.
Show me the mommy's girl.

Show me the car's driver.
Show me the driver's car.

Show me the captain's ship.
Show me the ship's captain.

*Negative/affirmative statements.* In the early stages of language development, it is not clear whether children are able to process negation when it is embedded in a sentence and attached to the auxiliary verb. Very often, in fact, the aspect of negation is contracted with the auxiliary, is unstressed, and is not very noticeable. It is very easy, and often likely, for the young child simply to overlook the addition of the phonemic element in a contraction such as *can't.*

*Examples:*

Show me: The doll can close her eyes.
Show me: The doll can't close her eyes.

Show me: The doll is standing.
Show me: The doll is not standing.
Show me: The doll isn't standing.

Show me: The dog has a bone.
Show me: The dog doesn't have a bone.

*Negative affirmative questions:* In this task, which is similar to the previous one, the child is presented with *wh-* questions rather than statements.

*Examples:*

What can you eat?
What can't you eat?

What can the girl wear?
What can't the girl wear?

What do you play with?
What don't you play with?

*Singular/plural with noun and verb inflections:* Even though the noun inflection for plurality appears early in language development, the verb inflection for third person singular appears much later. In singular and plural sentences in the third person such as, "The dog barks," and, "The dogs bark," the inflection occurs on the verb for the singular and on the noun for the plural.

*Examples:*

(Two boy dolls lying down. Demonstrate *walking*.)

Show me: The boy walks.
Show me: The boys walk.

(Two toy dogs. Demonstrate *jumping*.)

Show me: The dog jumps.
Show me: The dogs jump.

*Adjectival modification.* In a noun phrase, an adjective can be used to modify or alter the meaning of the head noun in the noun phrase. This applies to only the head noun of the phrase in which the adjective appears. So, in the sentence, "The little girl hit the boy," the adjective *little* applies only to the girl and provides no information about the object or *boy*. This seems quite simple, but often children in the middle stage of language development confuse the modification issue if the subject and the object of a sentence both are modified by adjectives.

*Examples:*

Show me: The little girl has a big doll.
Show me: The big girl has a little doll.

Put the round peg in the square hole.
Put the square peg in the round hole.

Show me the red dress with buttons.
Show me the dress with red buttons.

*Negative affix.* In the previous tasks, negation was dealt with on the level of sentence negation. Another type of negation is communicated through the use of affixes and is an inflection of only the word to which the affix is attached. Some such affixes that are negative are *un-*, *mis-* and *dis-*. The most familiar and earliest negative affix to appear is *un-* as in *untied.* In assessing negative affix, the clinician must determine whether the child learned words such as *tied* and *untied* as separate vocabulary items instead of learning the use of the affix to denote negation.

*Examples:*

Show me: The blocks are piled.
Show me: The blocks are unpiled.
Show me: The blocks are not piled.

Show me: The boxes are opened.
Show me: The boxes are not opened.
Show me: The boxes are unopened.

*Reflexivization.* Reflexives such as, "I looked at myself in the mirror," appear relatively late in language development. An earlier form that often appears is the object case pronoun instead of the reflexive pronoun in sentences like, "I saw me."

*Examples:*

Show me: Mommy washed her.
Show me: Mommy washed herself.

Show me: Billy hit him.
Show me: Billy hit himself.

Show me: The cat licked her.
Show me: The cat licked herself.

*Comparatives.* Another late appearing construction is the comparative, no doubt making its appearance only after the child has internalized the concept of comparison. As with the negative affix, the clinician must take care that some comparative words such as *more* and *less* have not been learned as separate vocabularly items that are synonymous with *big* and *little*. It would probably be advisable to avoid testing such words and to concentrate on comparative adjectives with *-er* suffixes.

*Examples:*

Give me a red stick shorter than a blue stick.
Give me a red stick longer than a blue stick.

Give me a short stick wider than a long stick.
Give me a short stick narrower than a long stick.

Show me the big box.
Show me the bigger box.

*Passives.* Passive sentences are those in which the normal word order of subject-verb-object is reversed. Thus, "The boy hit the girl," becomes, "The girl is hit by the boy." The two sentences are equivalent in meaning even with the reversal. The passive is another late appearing construction in language development and is often not fully comprehended until the child is about 4 years old. Younger children will often react to passive sentences as if they were active sentences, ignoring everything but the supposed subject-verb-object. In the sentence above, a child might focus upon, "The girl (is) hit (by) the boy," and interpret the sentence as if the words in parentheses were not present.

*Examples:*

Show me: The cat is chased by the dog.
Show me: The dog is chased by the cat.

Show me: The girl is washed by the boy.
Show me: The boy is washed by the girl.

*Self-embedded sentences.* One of the most interesting things about languages is that sentences can be of almost infinite length. One way that this is achieved is by "opening" the sentence and adding additional sentences of constituents to it. Consider the sentence, "The woman drove the car." One can insert another sentence, "The woman has a large dog," and produce the finished sentence, "The woman who has a large dog drove the car." In addition, one can insert the sentence, "The dog chased the cat," and produce, "The woman who has a large dog that chased the cat drove the car." There is no need to belabor the point, but this type of embedding can go on forever, as in the familiar nursery rhyme, "This is the House That Jack Built."

*Examples:*

(Use dolls and demonstrate *hitting* and *falling*.)

Show me: The boy that the girl hit fell down.
Show me: The girl that the boy hit fell down.

Show me: The cat that the dog chased jumped.
Show me: The dog that the cat chased jumped.

Show me: The cat that chased the dog jumped.
Show me: The dog that chased the cat jumped.

## Assessment of Language Production

In this section assessment techniques and procedures are discussed for the evaluation of (a) the oral speech mechanism, (b) articulatory proficiency, (c) syntax, and (d) semantics. Although the interrelatedness of comprehension and production and of syntax and semantics should be reemphasized, for purposes of discussing assessment, it is necessary to separate and dichotomize what are highly integrated aspects of language.

**Assessment of the Oral Speech Mechanism.** Assessment of the speech mechanism should encompass the examination of structure and function. All too often speech pathologists perform a speech mechanism examination in a ritualistic, perfunctory manner simply because they were taught in their training programs that such an examination is always done. However, if the clinician does not know the range of normalcy in oral anatomy and physiology, he or she can gain nothing from looking in children's mouths or asking them to say "puh-tuh-kuh" as fast as they can.

The examination should be systematic and rapid, which requires a considerable amount of practice. The clinician should use a process such as that outlined in this section to provide systematization and should take every opportunity to perfect his or her technique and observational skills. The proposed process, offered in a checklist format (Figure 5.2), is adapted from Sanders (1972) and provides for examination of both the structure of the speech mechanism and the function of the speech organs.

The results of the oral speech mechanism examination should provide the clinician with information related to the adequacy of the child's speech mechanism for the production of speech. In such an examination we do not usually find dramatic deviations of the oral structures that can be conclusively related to specific speech deviations, because most people are able to compensate for a number of structural irregularities. As a result we find that if the speaker can produce a sound correctly in some context, particularly in connected speech, the observed structural irregularities that he or she may have cannot be highly significant. However, we cannot overlook the

## FIGURE 5.2. A Checklist for the Peripheral Speech Mechanism Examination

I. *The Speech Mechanism at Rest and in Passive Motion*

A. General Body Position

1. Sitting Balance

______ Good, with head erect

______ Poor (see below)

______ Chest "collapsed"

______ Head and shoulders forward

______ Flattened upper rib cage

______ Must be held in position by assistive devices

2. Head Balance

______ Good

______ Poor (see below)

______ Involuntary movements; tremors

______ Turning to one side

______ Unable to lift in supine or prone position

______ Total body extensor tonus in supine position

______ Total body flexor tonus in prone position

3. Tonic Neck Reflex

______ Absent

______ Present

B. General Configuration and Muscular Control

1. Facial Symmetry

______ Normal

______ Abnormal (see below)

______ Facial muscles droop on one side (specify) ____________

______ One eye droops (specify) ________________________

______ Facial musculature pulled to one side (specify) ________

________________________________________________

______ Absence of naso-labial line on one side (specify) ______

________________________________________________

______ Greater retraction of one side of mouth (specify) ______

________________________________________________

______ Mandible pulls to one side (specify) ________________

**FIGURE 5.2.** continued

2. Feature Configuration

______ Normal

______ Abnormal (see below)

______ Unusual slant of palpebral fissures of the eye

______ Round flabby facies

______ Protruding lips

______ Rigid smile

______ Protruded, retruded, or underdeveloped mandible (check)

______ Scarred upper lip

3. Mouth

______ Normal

______ Abnormal (see below)

______ Open with tongue protruding

______ Drooling

______ Mouth breathing

4. Facial Musculature

______ Normal

______ Abnormal (see below)

______ Involuntary movement (specify)______________________

______ Primitive or infantile lip or tongue reflexes

______ Lip and tongue movement toward the side of the mouth, if stroked

______ Reflexive sucking

______ Reflexive pursing of the mouth when lips are tapped

______ Reflexive biting

5. Thoracic and Abdominal Musculature

______ Normal

______ Abnormal (see below)

______ Movement of the upper thoracic area during breathing

______ Evidence of opposition breathing

______ Resting breathing rate (specify) ______________________

______ Irregular breathing pattern

______ Stridorous noises during breathing

**FIGURE 5.2.** continued

II. *Voluntary Muscle Control During Speech*

A. Coordination of the Articulators During Speech

1. Range and Motion of Articulation Muscles

______ Adequate

______ Poor (see below)

______ Cannot move and shape articulators for phonemes that are

______ labial

______ labial-dental

______ lingua-dental

______ lingua-alveolar

______ lingua-palatal

______ nasal

______ glottal

2. Muscles of Respiration, Phonation, and Velopharyngeal Closure

______ Good

______ Poor (see below)

______ Difficulty initiating phonation during exhalation

______ Jaw thrust when initiating phonation

______ Nasal emission of air during speech

______ Inadequate velopharyngeal closure for plosive and fricative consonants

______ General incoordination of all muscles during speech

B. Phonation and Resonance

1. Pitch

______ Good

______ Poor (see below)

______ Too high

______ Too low

______ Pitch breaks

2. Intensity

______ Good

______ Poor (specify) ______________________________

3. Quality

______ Good

**FIGURE 5.2.** continued

_____ Poor (see below)

- _____ Hoarse
- _____ Breathy
- _____ Nasal
- _____ Denasal
- _____ Glottal "fry"
- _____ Diplophonia
- _____ Other (specify) ____________________

III. *Voluntary Muscle Control During Nonspeech Activities*

A. Mandible

_____ Good

_____ Poor (see below)

- _____ Cannot open and close easily on cue
- _____ Temporamandibular facet slip
- _____ Cannot click teeth together at the rate of two times per second

B. Lips

_____ Good

_____ Poor (see below)

- _____ Cannot purse and retract lips easily on cue
- _____ Cannot purse and retract at the rate of two times per second
- _____ Diminished mobility of upper lip due to scarring or tightness
- _____ Cannot show teeth by raising upper lip and depressing lower lip

C. Tongue

_____ Good

_____ Poor (see below)

- _____ Cannot protrude and retract easily on cue
- _____ Cannot elevate and depress to reach just beyond vermilion border of lips
- _____ Cannot lateralize smoothly
- _____ Cannot lateralize at the rate of two cycles per second
- _____ Involuntary movements when protruded for 3 to 4 seconds

**FIGURE 5.2.** continued

______ "Wave-like" movements

______ Deviation to one side during protrusion (specify) ______

______ Cannot point the tip

______ Cannot alternately narrow and flatten the blade

______ Cannot touch specific locations on the lips when stimulated

______ Thrust between the teeth during swallowing

______ Does not fit well in oral cavity (specify) ______

D. Dental Occlusion

______ Good

______ Poor (see below)

______ Obvious malocclusion

______ Space between incisors when molars are occluded

______ Maxillary arch lies within mandibular arch

______ Missing, extra, misplaced, or tilted teeth (specify) ______

______

E. Palate

______ Good

______ Poor (see below)

______ High and vaulted or low and flattened (check)

______ Evidence of a repaired or unrepaired cleft

______ Inadequate movement of palate and posterior pillars during production of /a/

______ Inadequate oral air pressure using an oral manometer

______ Inadequate fit of a speech appliance

F. Larynx and Muscles of Respiration

______ Good

______ Poor (see below)

______ Cannot sustain phonation for 10–15 seconds

______ Undue tension in neck muscles during phonation

______ Undue elevation of thyroid cartilage during phonation

______ Phonation during inhalation

In most cases the oral speech mechanism examination may be conducted as shown above. However, with some very young, severely mentally retarded, or severely neuromuscularly involved children, the examination may have to be conducted on a vegetative or emotional level. The following points should be checked:

**FIGURE 5.2.** continued

I. Vegetative Level

A. Biting, Chewing, and Swallowing

______ Adequate

______ Poor (see below)

______ Cannot open mouth to receive food

______ Does not use teeth to bite and chew

______ Accomplishes mastication by forward protrusion and elevation of tongue against palate

______ Cannot lateralize tongue to move food to chewing edge of teeth

______ Cannot use tongue to retrieve food from lip corners

______ Tongue thrust in swallowing

______ Tips head back to swallow

______ Chokes easily on soft foods

B. Drinking

______ Adequate

______ Poor (see below)

______ Tips head back to swallow when drinking from cup

______ Liquid escapes from nose

______ Cannot hold lips around a straw

______ Cannot develop negative pressure to drink from straw

C. Range of Motion in Eating

______ Adequate

______ Poor (see below)

______ Cannot feel bits of cracker or peanut butter placed on the lip or between the teeth and lips and retrieve them with the tongue

______ Cannot elevate tongue to retrieve bits of food placed behind the upper teeth or on the palate

______ Cannot protrude, point, or narrow tongue to lick lollipop held in front of mouth

II. Emotional Level

______ Adequate (in crying, laughing, smiling, showing fear or anger, etc.)

______ Poor (see below)

______ Does not retract lips in smiling

______ Does not open mouth to laugh

**FIGURE 5.2.** continued

______ Does not cup or thin the tongue

______ Does not elevate the soft palate

______ Does not sustain phonation

______ Other (from previous checklist items) ______________

Adapted, with permission, from *Procedure Guides for Evaluation of Speech and Language Disorders in Children*, 4th ed., by Lois Joan Sanders, 1979, Danville, IL: Interstate.

possibility that some inadequacy of the oral mechanism may account for, or contribute to, the speaker's inability to articulate proficiently. The clinician can teach some children with high, arched palates who have /r/ distortions to produce the /r/ correctly by artificially lowering the palate height (using chewing gum) and then, through a series of approximations, teaching the child to make the /r/ when the palate is allowed to return to its usual height by using less gum to occlude the space between the tongue and the palate.

**Assessment of Speech Sound Production.** To plan an articulation therapy program, as in other areas of language therapy, it is not enough simply to know that the child has an articulation error. The clinician must be concerned with four basic areas:

- What sounds are produced incorrectly? What are the characteristics of the misarticulations? These points are discussed in the following section (Phonemic Analysis) and are the points covered by most articulation tests.
- How does the child misarticulate? This question is related to the oral speech mechanism examination, because it centers around the specific muscle patterns that produce the misarticulations.
- What is the variability of the misarticulation? Under what acoustic or contextual conditions does the misarticulation vary?
- Why does the child misarticulate? Can any related deficiencies be identified, such as poor speech sound discrimination, structural anomalies, inadequate neuromuscular abilities, or inappropriate linguistic models? Answers to all of these questions may not be possible, but because children with so-called "functional" articulation problems often have syntactic and semantic disorders as well, it is worthwhile to investigate the full parameters of what may look like a simple speech problem.

*Phonemic analysis.* Almost any standard articulation test will suffice to answer the first diagnostic question, "What sounds are misarticulated and what are the characteristics of the misarticulation?" The results of such a test will reveal (a) which sounds are in error, (b) what type of misarticulations are present (omissions, substitutions, or distortions), (c) where the errors occur (in initial, medial, or final position), and (d) in some tests, where the place of articulation is (e.g., labial, dental, alveolar). Some clinicians have been taught to make their own articulation tests, but with the number of good instruments on the market, there seems little benefit to be gained from such a time-consuming and tedious task. No doubt it is a useful exercise to make beginning students more aware of phonemes and to enhance their own listening skills, but because phonemic analysis is so well-covered by commercial tests, examiner-constructed tests will not be further discussed.

*Kinetic analysis.* Van Riper (1963) describes a way to assess articulation disorders that he terms *kinetic analysis*. This procedure investigates what specifically a child is doing to produce the phonemes in a defective manner. To conduct such an analysis, the clinician must draw on Powers' (1957) description of the necessary motor requirements for accurate sound production. She suggests that there must be precision of movement in terms of placement of structures, direction of movements, amount of contact surface, and the shape of the contact between structures. Articulatory movements must also be made at the appropriate speed, they must be made with enough energy or pressure, and there must be synergy of the sequential movements necessary for connected speech.

To conduct the kinetic analysis, three methods may be employed. First, the clinician can ask the child to tell what he or she is doing. This is probably the least fruitful approach, because even adult clients can seldom describe how they are producing a given sound. As children and adults progress in therapy, they are better able to describe phonemic production, but they still have difficulty describing anything more complex than whether the tip of the tongue is elevated. The second method is to watch what the child is doing. For example, does the tongue protrude between the incisors when the /s/ or /z/ is produced? Does the mandible shift to one side when sibilants are uttered? If either of these two phenomena are observed, it is likely that a major reason for a central or lateral lisp has been discovered, and a central focus for therapy has been established. If the reader has any doubt on this score, he or she should try producing the word *some* with the tongue protruding between the central incisors during the production of the initial /s/. The result will be a classic central lisp—*thum* instead of *some*. The third method of kinetic analysis is probably the best. Taking advantage of their trained ears and knowledge of motor phonetics, clinicians can attempt to duplicate in their own production what the child is doing. By listening carefully and experimenting with the placement of the articulators, the clinician can learn to make the child's error, providing a basis for altering the child's production in an objective, systematic fashion.

The kinetic analysis may reveal obvious motor disorders; indeed, such an analysis could be incorporated into the initial stages of the oral speech mechanism examination. Regardless, the clinician must learn as much as possible about motor phonetics to understand the motor elements of phonemic production. Only through such knowledge will the clinician become an accurate observer or imitator of the movements of speech production.

*Sources of variability.* Identifying misarticulated phonemes and determining how the phonemes are being produced is only half of the diagnostic task. The clinician must also investigate the circumstances that may improve the child's articulatory production. Because inconsistency of production is an important clinical sign, we must discover whether children ever produce their error sounds correctly. If the error sounds are produced correctly, even only occasionally, we can assume children have the normal capability of improving their articulation. It is a good prognostic sign and provides a starting point of therapy. Four types of variability are discussed in the following section: connected speech, stimulability, key words, and deep testing.

1. *Connected speech.* The major problem with articulation tests is that they are designed to evoke single words, and that is not how we speak—not even the most taciturn of us. Speech is a dynamic, overlapping, incredibly swift, flowing activity. If one has good ears and listens carefully, one can distinguish individual phonemes in the flow, but each of these phonemes is influenced by the phonemes which precede and follow it. This phenomenon is known as *coarticulation* and may extend across four or five phonemes. Because of this, a complete assessment of a child's articulation cannot be limited to the examination of single words but must include an evaluation of spontaneous, connected speech that will more accurately reflect habitual articulation behavior.

Connected speech samples can be elicited in a number of ways, such as conversing, retelling a story, narrating a recent event, reading a paragraph, and so on. The speech sample can be tape recorded and an articulation inventory done at the clinician's leisure. The results of the analysis of the speech sample should be compared with the results of an articulation test to determine whether there is inconsistency in phonemic production under the two differing conditions and, if so, what the characteristics of the variability are.

2. *Stimulability.* In many cases, children are able to imitate the correct production of their error sounds by imitating their clinician's productions. Even if the production is not truly accurate, there may be movement away from the error toward the correct production. Testing for stimulability is a feature of several articulation tests, but further testing by the clinician should be done to determine whether children can imitate correct production of their error sounds on single words, in isolation, in nonsense syllables,

and in limited connected speech. If the child is stimulable, there are usually no significant obstacles that would prevent eventual acquisition of the sound. Results of stimulability assessment also give the clinician a starting point for therapy when a child produces a number of defective sounds. The sounds that are most stimulable are the ones that should be corrected first.

3. *Key words.* It is not unusual to find that children will produce correctly their error sounds in certain words, often words that are discovered only in conversation with them. It is valuable to discover such key words because, as Van Riper (1963) says,

> . . . they provide for the person a model in his own mouth for the sound we seek to teach him. We can use these key words to help us perceive the characteristics of the standard sound, both acoustic cues and the postures and movements required for their production. They can be used in discriminating error words from normally spoken words. (p. 231)

Van Riper's statement is important not only with reference to key words but to any condition under which a child is able to produce a sound correctly.

4. *Deep testing.* The phenomenon of coarticulation (i.e., the fact that each phoneme produced by a speaker is influenced by the phonemic context in which it occurs) is discussed above. Most articulation tests provide for only a superficial evaluation of the many possible phonemic contexts in which a child's misarticulated sound may occur. McDonald (1964) developed the *Deep Test of Articulation* to assess a child's misarticulation in all possible phonemic contexts. The *Test of Articulation Performance–Diagnostic* (Bryant & Bryant, 1983) also provides for deep testing, although in a more limited fashion than the McDonald test. Deep testing need not be administered routinely during a diagnostic evaluation, but the clinician should use either the test or the procedure during the initial stages of therapy to determine the phonemic contexts in which a misarticulated sound is produced correctly, thereby providing a starting point for therapy.

*Linguistic analysis.* For some time, clinicians have observed that children with functional articulation disorders are also deficient in other language skills. Authors such as Compton (1970), Fisher and Logemann (1971), and McReynolds and Huston (1971) pointed out some time ago that individuals with articulation disorders do not simply have an incomplete, random system of phonemic production. Rather, a careful phonological analysis of the speech of such individuals reveals that in many cases logical and coherent principles underlie their idiosyncratic use of speech sounds. According to McReynolds and Huston (1971),

> when articulation errors occur, they may consist of a phoneme system organized differently from the adult phoneme system. The more the systems differ,

> the more severe the child's articulation problem. The child's system may be complete for the child and as lawful as the adult's but it is his own system, and his rules are at variance with the adult or the standard system. (pp. 155–156)

In terms of assessment, attention is shifted from the child's actual error sound to the underlying patterns that the errors follow. Clinicians may use one of the commercially available tests that include the dimension of distinctive feature analysis, such as the Fisher-Logeman or the TAP–D. Or clinicians may do their own analysis using the results of articulation assessment as described above and recording the data on a chart such as the one shown in Figure 5.3. The data to be recorded would be only correct productions, and the clinician would be able to determine quite easily which distinctive features the child is missing. The only features selected for analysis are the common ones of place of articulation, manner of articulation, and voicing. The results of such an analysis are shown in Figure 5.4. One might draw several conclusions with regard to a therapy program from these results.

The child whose correct productions are recorded in Figure 5.4 has only six correct phonemes—/m/, /p/, /b/, /t/, /d/, and /h/. For /k/, /t/ or /h/ was substituted; for /g/, /d/ and /h/ were substituted; for /θ/, /t/ was substituted; and for /ð/ and /n/, /d/ was substituted. All other phonemes were replaced by the voiceless, glottal /h/. Based on this information, the following suggestions for therapy could be made.

- Teach some of the features that classify sounds—for example, teach the feature of friction as it relates to changes at the place of articulation.
- Use words like *hip* and *ship* to show how meaning is changed when the place of articulation changes from the common /h/ to the lingua-palatal contrast. Enlarge the categories for the auditory discrimination of speech sounds.
- Do all types of auditory training exercises using the correct sounds and contrasts.
- Use tongue exercises to help explore the structures of the mouth and the variety of movements possible among articulators.

Other excellent presentations of phonological analysis procedures are available in addition to those already mentioned. Some of these approaches are the description of distinctive feature analysis by Pollack and Rees (1972), generative phonology by Schane (1973), and natural generative phonology by Ingram (1976). Shriberg and Kwiatkowski's (1980) natural process approach is particularly helpful in linking developmental phonology with syntax and semantics.

**Assessment of Syntactic Production.** Two general procedures are presented for the assessment of both syntactic and semantic production: the

**FIGURE 5.3. A Chart for the Analysis of Phonemic Errors Using a Distinctive Features Approach**

| | V | N-V | V | N-V | V | N-V | V | N-V | V | N-V | V | N-V | V | N-V |
|---|---|---|---|---|---|---|---|---|---|---|---|---|---|---|
| Glide | | | | | | | | | | | | | | |
| Semivowel | | | | | | | | | | | | | | |
| Nasal | | | | | | | | | | | | | | |
| Stop | | | | | | | | | | | | | | |
| Fricative | | | | | | | | | | | | | | |
| | Labial | | Labiodental | | Dental | | Alveolar | | Palatal | | Velar | | Glottal | |

V = voiced
N-V = non-voiced

**FIGURE 5.4. A Child's Articulation Performance.**

| | V | N-V | V | N-V | V | N-V | V | N-V | V | N-V | V | N-V | V | N-V |
|---|---|---|---|---|---|---|---|---|---|---|---|---|---|---|
| Glide | | | | | | | | | | | | | | |
| Semivowel | | | | | | | | | | | | | | |
| Nasal | m | | | | | | | | | | | | | |
| Stop | b | p | | | | | d | t | | | | | | |
| Fricative | | | | | | | | | | | | | | h |
| | Labial | | Labiodental | | Dental | | Alveolar | | Palatal | | Velar | | Glottal | |

V = voiced
N-V = non-voiced

language sample analysis and elicited production tasks. Readers should refer to the beginning of this chapter to refresh their memory regarding the procedures for securing a language sample and estimating the mean length of utterance (MLU). The first assessment is computing the MLU; the second is a distributional analysis. These are followed by de Villiers and de Villiers' (1973) stage assignments for Brown's 14 grammatical morphemes, an example of Miller's (1981) assessment profile, and finally, a series of elicitation techniques. For a variety of other techniques and procedures that can be used to assess syntactic production in depth, see Table 5.6 as suggested by Miller (1981).

*Distributional analysis.* A distributional analysis is a reorganization of the transcript of a language sample by specific utterance characteristics. Three types of segmentation of transcripts can be effected: by sentence length, by syntactic structure, and by number of utterances per speaking turn. The MLU will be clarified by a distributional analysis of sentence length. Ideally, variations in sentence length around the mean should exist but should not be extreme in their variance. A number of spuriously long sentences will significantly inflate the MLU and render it nonrepresentative. If the language sample consists of utterances that are all only one or two words in length, there may be a limitation in production due to functional problems in the oral speech mechanism. To analyze the distribution of sentence length, simply make a list of the utterances with one morpheme, two morphemes, three morphemes, and so on. By reviewing such a list the clinician can quickly determine whether the MLU seems to be representative.

Analyzing the distribution of syntactic structures in the language sample provides the clinician with a view of the structural variety within the sample. At the same time that the clinician is examining the specific structures produced, he or she may record the length of utterance associated with the structures. A very simple way to go about this type of analysis is to list the structures, the number of utterances in which each structure occurred, and the length of the utterances as shown below.

| Structural Analysis | Total Number of Utterances | MLU per Type of Structure |
|---|---|---|
| Noun phrase elaboration | | |
| Verb phrase elaboration | | |
| Noun inflections | | |
| Verb inflections | | |
| Yes/no questions | | |
| *Wh-* questions | | |
| Negation | | |

## TABLE 5.6. Procedures for In-Depth Analysis of Children's Syntactic Production

| Content | Procedure | Sample size | Range of use | Reference |
|---|---|---|---|---|
| Syntax | Developmental Sentence Types (DST) | 100 utterances | 22 months–6 years | Lee (1966) |
| | Developmental Sentence Analysis (DSS) | 50 complete sentences | 3–7 years | Lee (1974) |
| | Language Sampling, Analysis and Training (LSAT) | 100 utterances | 2–10 years | Tyack and Gottsleben (1974) |
| | Language Assessment, Remediation and Screening Procedure (LARSP) | 30 minutes<br>100–200 utterances | 22 months–5 years | Crystal, Fletcher & Garman (1976) |
| | Scale of Children's Clausal Development (SCCD) | Transcript of unspecified length | 18–40 months<br>1.5–5 years | Dever and Bauman (1974) |
| | *TALK*-Assessing Current Functioning | 6–8 pages (200+ utterances) | | Dever (1978) |
| | Co-occurring and Restricted Structure Procedure (CORS) | Representative sample (usually requiring several samples in varying situations) | 1.5–5 years | Muma (1973) |
| | Linguistic Analysis of Speech Samples (LASS) | 75–100 utterances | 5–11 years | Engler, Hannah and Longhurst (1973) |
| | Assigning Structural Stage (ASS) | At least 50 utterances in at least two contexts | 18 months–7 years | Miller (1981) |

From *Assessing Language Production in Children: Experimental Procedures* (p. 30) by J. Miller, 1981, Austin, TX: PRO-ED. Reprinted by permission.

Structures that are produced within longer utterances or low frequency utterances may be found in the initial stages of acquisition.

The analysis of the distribution of utterances per speaking turn is not really related to syntactic production but is, instead, one way of assessing the more pragmatic level of language. Categorically, this analysis would be done at the same time that the other distributional analyses are done. See the Assessment of Pragmatics section later in this chapter for a discussion of this segmentation.

*de Villiers and de Villiers' 14 morpheme analysis.* Table 5.7 shows de Villiers and de Villiers' (1973) stage assignments for the 14 grammatical morphemes used by Brown (1973) in researching the stages of normal language

**TABLE 5.7. Stage Assignments for 14 Grammatical Morphemes**

| Stage | Morpheme | Example |
|---|---|---|
| II | *-ing* | Me playing. |
| | plural | That books. |
| | *in* | Cookie Monster in there. |
| III | *on* | Doggie on car. |
| | possessive | Mommy's shoe. |
| V | regular past | He walked. |
| | irregular past | She came.<br>We went. |
| | regular third person singular | It jumps.<br>She plays. |
| | articles *a, the* | That's a puppy.<br>Here is the paper. |
| | contractible copula *be* | Here's my coat.<br>Those are my crayons. |
| V+ | contractible auxiliary *be* | They're playing.<br>I am coming. |
| | uncontractible copula *be* | Who's here? I *am*. |
| | uncontractible auxiliary *be* | Who's playing? I *am*. |
| | irregular third person singular | She has.<br>He does. |

Adapted from "A Cross-Sectional Study of the Acquisition of Grammatical Morphemes in Child Speech" by J. de Villiers and P. de Villiers, 1973, *Journal of Psycholinguistic Research, 2,* 267–268. Reprinted by permission.

development. The clinician will need some type of worksheet for recording the 14 morpheme analysis, and the one developed by Miller (1981) can serve as a prototype (see Figure 5.5). Whatever kind of worksheet the clinician designs, it will need to have space for recording several types of information, as follows:

- a space for each morpheme
- a space to indicate the number of the utterance in which the morpheme is present
- a way of indicating that the morpheme is obligatory in the specific utterance (Miller uses a check to indicate the presence of a morpheme and a minus to indicate the absence of it in the obligatory context.)
- space for recording the percentage of occurrence, which is obtained by dividing the number of morphemes present in one realm, such as plurals, by the number of obligatory contexts

The reader should note that the terms *contractible* and *uncontractible* refer to whether the verb can be contracted in Standard English, not to whether the child has or has not contracted the verb in his or her language sample. It makes no difference to the stage assignment for the child if he or she has said "I am going" or "I'm going." Uncontractible verbs are usually found in the sentence-final position and can never be correctly contracted. One may say "I am" in response to the question "Who's here?" but may not respond "I'm."

*Elicited production.* Elicited production is not to be confused with elicited imitation, which is an outright imitation by the child of the clinician's production. However, in elicited production the situation is structured so that the child is led into producing the desired oral response without the need for imitation. Elicitation techniques may be used for a variety of reasons: (a) when the clinician wishes to assess specific aspects of language, (b) when certain structures appear only infrequently in naturalistic settings, and (c) when time for assessment is limited. The following procedures for eliciting specific structures are taken from Bellugi (in Slobin, 1967) and are considered appropriate for children aged 3 through 12 years.

1. *Interrogation.* Using dolls or puppets, tell the child to "Ask the doll ________________," using the indirect form of the question (e.g., "Ask the doll what she wants"). Try to focus on eliciting questions that are structurally difficult or rare. The verb phrase can be anything that the clinician feels is appropriate to the situation.

**FIGURE 5.5. Worksheet for 14 Morpheme Analysis**

| Stage | Morpheme | Utterances | Scoring |
|---|---|---|---|
| II | -ing | | |
| II | plural | 49) blocks | ✓ — 100% |
| II | in | 4) in<br>38) in | ✓<br>✓<br>100% |
| III | on | | |
| III | possessive | | |
| V | irregular past | | |
| V | article | 18) the<br>40) a | ✓<br>✓<br>100% |
| V | regular past | | |
| V | regular third person singular | 1) stands<br>52) comes | ✓<br>come<br>50% |
| V | contractible copula <u>be</u> | 4) 's<br>19) 's<br>21) is<br>22) is<br>28) 's<br>36) 's<br>49) 're<br>50) is | –<br>✓<br>✓<br>✓<br>–<br>✓<br>–<br>✓<br>63% |
| V+ | contractible auxiliary <u>be</u> | | |
| V+ | irregular third person singular | 38) does | ✓ — 100% |
| V+ | uncontractible auxiliary <u>be</u> | | |
| V+ | uncontractible copula <u>be</u> | | |

From *Assessing Language Production in Children: Experimental Procedures* (p. 30) by J. Miller, 1981, Austin, TX: PRO-ED. Reprinted by permission.

*Examples:*

*Vary the interrogative word*

What she wants
Where she put it
When she'll do it
How she got it

*Vary the noun phrase and the auxiliary verb*

What she can do
What I might have
What they will have been doing
What the boy is supposed to see

*Vary with negative*

Why she doesn't help
Why I can't do it
Why they aren't here yet

*Vary the subject and object*

Who pushed John
Who did John push

Instead of using dolls or puppets with older children, it would probably be more appropriate to bring into the room a third person and phrase the command, "Ask Mr. Smith ________________" (e.g., "Ask him what his name is," "Ask Mr. Smith why he is here," etc.).

2. *Tag questions.* The production of tag questions ("He did it, didn't he?") appears relatively late in children's language development. It follows a declarative sentence and generally asks for confirmation of the statement. Other common forms are: "He's here, right?" "Give me the book, okay?" and "Huh?" after a statement. These less elegant productions usually occur in children's speech well before the true tag questions.

Tag questions are of particular interest, because the form of the tag is explicitly determined by the syntax of the sentence it follows. According to Bellugi (in Slobin, 1967), the following processes are involved in the formation of tags:

1. The speaker must pronominalize the noun phrase subject of the sentence.
2. The speaker must locate (and perhaps supply *do* or the full form of) the first auxiliary verb of the main clause of the sentence.
3. The speaker negates the auxiliary of the sentence if it is affirmative but not if it is negative.

4. Finally, the speaker must invert the auxiliary verb and the pronominalized noun phrase.

As the reader can see, the speaker must follow a very complex procedure in producing tag questions. The procedure for assessing children's ability to produce such structures can provide information about their ability to locate the subject of a sentence, pronominalize nouns and noun phrases, handle conjoined noun phrases, define sentence negation, handle auxiliaries that they may not produce, locate the first element of an auxiliary verb, handle subject-verb agreement and tense agreement, define the subject and auxiliary of an imperative sentence, and so on.

The examiner can begin to elicit tag questions using a set of instructions such as those suggested by Miller (1981):

> Suppose I want to say something, and I'm not really sure about it. I might say: "The sun is shining today," and then, I might add: "Isn't it?" We're going to play a game like that. I'll say something, and you can add the last part, like this. I say, "That alligator can bite very hard," and you say, "_______________." (p. 146)

The range of information available to the examiner through this elicitation procedure is shown in Table 5.8 adapted from Bellugi (in Miller, 1981).

3. *Negativization.* In Slobin (1967), Bellugi discusses elicitation procedures that can be used to assess children's ability to produce a variety of negatives, which are generally more easily elicited than some of the other structures discussed. Basically, the child is asked to provide the negative of a sentence that is supplied by the examiner, who may use a variety of techniques to initiate the process. It probably would be easiest to begin by asking the child to imitate sentences, thus giving him or her a clue as to what patterns are expected and what patterns are beyond the child's capacity.

The examiner gives the following instructions: "I'll say something and then you say the opposite. I'll say, 'The boy can run,' and you say, 'The boy can't run.'" The various types of negatives that can be assessed are given below with sample sentences:

*Vary Auxiliary*

| | |
|---|---|
| The boy can run. | The boy __________. |
| The dish will break. | The dish __________. |
| The girl is crying. | The girl __________. |
| The cat went outside. | The cat __________. |

## TABLE 5.8. Examples of the Range of Information Available in Tag Questions (Bellugi, in Slobin, 1967)

**Affirmative/negative interaction**

I will do it.
I won't do it.

He could come.
He couldn't come.

**Be and have**

It's been done now.
It's coming now.

John's tired.
John's finished his lunch.

They're doing it.
I was going.

They were annoyed.
I'm coming.

**First element of auxiliary**

He could have done it.
I will have been swimming since this morning.
They would have been coming anyway.

**Tense agreement**

I go there often.
I went there yesterday.

He walked farther.
He walks frequently.

**Location of grammatical subject**

The girl pushed the boy.
The boy was pushed by the girl.

John and you played together.
Three boys and a girl are playing together.

**Definition of sentence negation**

He came here.
He never came.

He is unhappy.
He is happy.

I saw the boy who didn't go to school.
The boy who didn't go to school was fishing.

Nobody likes me.
Everybody likes me.

They have no sense.
They have little sense.

**Modal auxiliaries**

I could have found it.
They should arrive soon.
He will ask us.
She can do it.

**Subject and auxiliary of imperatives**

Help me find this book.
Sit down.
Come here.

***Do* as auxiliary verb**

I need some cookies.
You see the truck.

**Subject-verb agreement**

I hit the ball.
He hits the ball.

You throw the stone.
John throws the stone.

**Pronominalization**

John came home early.
Sue is running.
The boys are playing.
The chair tipped over.

Both of them did it.
The two of us want some.

John and Bill played together.
John and I played together.

Yesterday after we came home from a long walk, the little girl came out to greet us.
I know where the boy is hiding.
The boys who jumped over the fence in my neighbors' yard ran away.

**Limit on applicability of tag**

Who finished this?

From *Assessing Language Production in Children: Experimental Procedures* (p. 147) by J. Miller, 1981, Austin, TX: PRO-ED. Reprinted by permission.

*Negative with Indefinite*

The girl ate some soup. The girl __________.

He wants some cookies. ________________.

Someone saw her. ________________.

Someone is coming in. ________________.

*Imperatives*

Come in here. ________________.

Sit down over there. ________________.

*Multi-Propositional Sentences*

I saw the cat who came. ________________.

She asked him to do it. ________________.

Someone wants him to take some. ________________.

Why does she do that? ________________.

4. *Reflexivization.* Reflexivization is a grammatical structure that can be elicited in only a limited way. In English, whenever the subject and the object of certain verbs are the same, the object is reflexivized. In children's speech, and indeed in the speech of adults in some geographic regions of the country, the intermediate stage of reflexivization is often encountered. "I made me a glass of tea" is heard in place of "I made myself a glass of tea."

To begin eliciting reflexives, the examiner should have several sets of pictures illustrating the same action being performed on the individual represented and on another individual. For example, in one picture a girl may be washing her face, and in another picture she may be washing her doll's face. The pictures are presented to the child with the accompanying sentences: "The girl washed the doll." "The girl washes herself." Because reflexives may be difficult to elicit, the examiner should be prepared with several sets of pictures to assist the child in setting the appropriate pattern. Some of the sentences that the examiner might use to elicit reflexives are

*Pronominalization*

The girl washed ________(herself)________.

The boy cut ________(himself)________.

The girl looked at ________(herself)________.

I see ________(myself)________.

*Imperatives*

Behave _______(yourself)_______.

Protect _______(yourself)_______.

It should be noted that according to English rules of grammar, reflexivization does not occur outside of sentence boundaries. Prepositions are reflexivized; therefore, one cannot reflexivize the subject of the main clause, as in "I want her to take care of (herself, not myself)" or "Mary wanted John to help her (himself, not herself)."

**Assessment of Semantic Production.** In assessing semantics it is important to distinguish between semantics and other developmental functions, such as cognition, and to distinguish between semantics and syntax and pragmatics. One may consider the underlying concepts that children acquire as cognition and the means for expressing these concepts in words as semantics. For the purposes of this discussion, we will limit the subject to children's expressions of meanings through language. The distinction between semantics and syntax or semantics and pragmatics is very elusive because of the generous overlaps among them. For example, many of the early semantic roles that researchers have investigated (e.g., agent, action, object) are both semantic and syntactic, because they characterize the meaning of the words that fill the slots in the sentence and they represent something about their grammatic function as well. Agents, a semantic characterization, are almost always sentence subjects, a grammatic representation. Consistent word order in a child's speech reflects that the child knows these roles fulfill more than meaningful categorization. And children seem to know that these categories must be combined in a certain structure or sequence to express the desired meaning—a grammatic sequence. Bloom and Lahey (1978) refer to these early semantic role combinations as *semantic-syntactic relations*. In assessing semantics, the specifically semantic component of the grammar will be extracted as much as possible.

As mentioned above, semantics and pragmatics overlap to such a degree that it is often impossible to separate the meaning of a sentence from its use. If I say, "Can you hand me that book?" the literal meaning of my sentence ("Are you able to hand me the book?") is not what I probably intended you to understand.

For several reasons, this section presents a very limited introduction to the area of investigating a child's use of semantic knowledge. First, many semantic taxonomies have been developed and presented in the developmental literature, but very little work has been done in applying these taxonomies to clinical populations as assessment tools. Second, and more important, there is not a clear developmental sequence for the acquisition of semantic production beyond the period of Brown's stages I or II. What is presented here is a framework for thinking about semantic development.

In 1973, de Villiers and de Villiers proposed a distinction between referential meaning and relational meaning in their discussion of semantic development. Referential meaning concerns the one-to-one link between words and the objects for which they stand. Relational meaning has to do with the connections between and among concepts, words, and sentences.

*Referential meaning.* In assessment, referential meaning is investigated primarily through an analysis of the child's use of individual words. Two types of analyses are suggested by Miller (1981): (a) the type-token ration and (b) semantic field analysis. The type-token ration, developed by Templin (1957), provides the examiner with an index of lexical diversity. The procedure used by Templin calculates vocabulary usage based on the number of different words produced by the child in a 50-utterance sample and the total number of words in the sample. The relationship between these two measures is derived by dividing the total number of words used into the total number of different words used, as shown below:

$$\text{Type-Token Ration} = \frac{\text{Total Number Different Words}}{\text{Total Number Words}}$$

Templin, who studied the type-token ratios (TTR) of 480 children, reported ratios of approximately .50 occurring consistently across all age groups, sex groups, and socioeconomic status groups. Because of this consistency, the TTR is a remarkably useful measure.

Type-token ratios are easy to compute from transcripts. The following procedures for the computation (Templin, 1957) should be followed as closely as possible.

I. *Utterance sample*

Templin employed McCarthy's (1930) procedures in collecting speech samples. She used pictures and toys as stimulus materials and recorded 50 consecutive utterances. Utterance boundaries were determined by what were called "a natural break in the verbalization of the child."[1]

II. *Rules for counting numbers of words*

A. Contractions of subject and predicate like *it's* or *I'll* are counted as two words.

[1]From *Certain Language Skills in Children* (Institute of Child Welfare Monograph Series No. 26) (p. 15) by M. Templin, 1957, Minneapolis, MN: University of Minnesota Press. Reprinted by permission.

B. Contractions of the verb and the negative such as *isn't* are counted as one word.
C. Each part of a verbal combination is counted as a separate word; thus, *have been playing* is counted as three words.
D. Hyphenated and compound words are counted as one word.
E. Expressions that function as one word, such as *oh boy, all right,* etc. are counted as one word.
F. Articles—*a, an, the*—are counted as one word.
G. Bound morphemes (such as *-ness, -ly,* etc.) and noun and verb inflections are not counted as separate words.[2]

III. *Computing the Type-Token Ratio*

A. Identify 50 consecutive utterances from the sample, preferably the middle 50.
B. Count the total number of words expressed using the rules given above under II.
C. Count the total number of different words produced.
D. Divide the total number of different words by the total number of words produced. The result is the TTR.[3]

The second type of referential semantic assessment is the semantic field analysis, which provides the examiner with another way of investigating the range of a child's vocabulary. For this particular analysis, there is no standardized procedure. Instead, the examiner must create a set of meaning categories for the words that appear in the transcript of the speech sample. Noun categories might be animals, people, vehicles, toys, and so on; verb categories could be movement, existence, desire, and so on; and adverb or adjective categories could be duration (*long, short*), temporal sequence (*first, last*), manner (*hard, loud*), and distance (*near, far*).

The words in the transcript are classified according to the various categories created, and the examiner then has some idea regarding the diversity and complexity of the child's vocabulary in terms of both the number of meaningful categories and the number of different words in each category. For example, if the categorical concepts are encoded by children who have low levels of structural development, the examiner could predict a discrepancy between their cognitive and linguistic performance.

*Relational meaning.* At least three levels of analysis of the semantics of relational meaning can be posited: intrasentence relations, intersentence relations, and contextual (or nonlinguistic) relations. The most extensively studied aspect of the semantics of relational meaning is intrasentence relations

---

[2]Ibid., p. 160.

[3]Ibid., p. 160.

(Bloom, 1973; Brown, 1970, 1973; Greenfield & Smith, 1976; and Schlesinger, 1971). It appears that children produce a rather restricted number of intrasentence relations in 2- to 3-word sentences even though they could produce a great many. Brown (1973) describes a set of common relations to look for in Stage I to II children, and Retherford, Schwartz, and Chapman (in Miller, 1981) present a scheme for coding the relations in a speech sample transcript, as shown in Figure 5.6.

Note that there are no developmental data for semantic role analysis for children above Stage II, and, therefore, analysis of children above that stage of development would be unreliable. The examiner who is well versed in the literature on semantic development could devise assessment procedures to evaluate some of the more complex semantic relations at the intrasentence level (e.g., conjunctions joining two propositions within one utterance, the content of requests, and the content of questions).

A number of intersentence and contextual relations, such as pronominal reference, deixis, discourse cohesion, and communicative intent, could be investigated by the examiner. However, there are very little developmental data in these areas, and they overlap so closely with pragmatics that it would be better not to consider them semantic functions. To summarize, semantic analyses can include the assessment of referential and relational meanings. While referential meaning is examined with regard to single words, relational meaning can be explored within a single sentence or between sentences.

## Assessment of Pragmatics

To reemphasize a major point regarding pragmatics and not, it is hoped, to belabor the point, language always occurs in a context, and all contexts are not the same. Implicit in this statement is the assumption that language production varies with the context in which it is produced. Although the research is not reviewed here, there is evidence that language varies with the communicative partner and within different physical contexts. For the interested reader, Gallagher (1983) presents a brief and lucid review of the literature.

An entirely new vocabulary must be learned to read the literature on pragmatics in childhood language. It is not within the parameters of the present book to present, define, and discuss this vocabulary or the many taxonomies of pragmatic function that have been developed. The decision was made to review briefly the work of Prutting and Kirchner (1983), Halliday (1975), and Dore (1975), because it seems that their work provides a framework for the examiner to develop assessment strategies.

## FIGURE 5.6. Definitions of the 21 Semantic Categories

**Action**[a] A perceivable movement or activity engaged in by an agent (animate or inanimate).

**Entity** (One-term utterances only) any labeling of the present person or object regardless of the occurrence or nature or action being performed on or by it.

**Entity** (Multi-term utterances only) The use of an appropriate label for a person or object in the absence of any action on it (with the exception of showing, pointing, touching, or grasping); or someone or something that caused or was the stimulus to the internal state specified by a state verb or any object or person that was modified by a possessive form. (**Entity** was used to code a possession if it met either of the preceding criteria).

**Locative** The place where an object or action was located or toward which it moved.

**Negation**[b] The impression of any of the following meanings with regard to someone or something, or an action or state: non-existence, rejection, cessation, denial, disappearance.

**Agent** The performer (animate or inanimate) of an action. Body parts and vehicles, when used in conjunction with action verbs, were coded **Agent**.

**Object** A person or thing (marked by the use of a noun or pronoun) that received the force of an action.

**Demonstrative** The use of demonstrative pronouns or adjectives, *this, that, these, those,* and the words *there, right there, here, see,* when stated for the purpose of pointing out a particular referent.

**Recurrence** A request for or comment on an additional instance or amount; the resumption of an event; or the reappearance of a person or object.

**Attribute** An adjectival description of the size, shape, or quality of an object or person; also, noun adjuncts which modified nouns for a similar purpose (e.g., *gingerbread* man).

**Possessor** A person or thing (marked by the use of a proper noun or pronoun) that an object was associated with or to which it belonged, at least temporarily.

**Adverbial**[c] Included in this category were the two subcategories of action/attribute and state/attribute.

**Action/Attribute** A modifier of an action indicating time, manner, duration, distance, or frequency. (Direction or place of action was separately coded as **Locative, Repetition** and **Recurrence**).

**State/Attribute** A modifier indicating time, manner, quality, or intensity of a state.

**Quantifier** A modifier that indicated amount or number or a person or object. Prearticles and indefinite pronouns such as *a piece of, lots of, any, every,* and *each* were included.

**State** A passive condition experienced by a person or object. This category implies involuntary behavior on the part of the **Experiencer**, in contrast to voluntary action performed by an **Agent**.

**Experiencer** Someone or something that underwent a given experience or mental state. Body parts, when used in conjunction with state verbs, were coded **Experiencer**.

**Recipient** One who received or was named as the recipient of an *object* (person or thing) from another.

**Beneficiary** One who benefited from or was named as the beneficiary of a specified action.

**Name** The labeling or request for naming of a person or thing using the utterance forms: *my (his, your,* etc.) *name is* ________ or *what's* ________ *name?*

**Created Object** Something created by a specific activity, for example, a *song* by singing, a *house* by building, a *picture* by drawing.

**Comitative** One who accompanied or participated with an agent in carrying out a specified activity.

**Instrument** Something that an **Agent** used to carry out or complete a specified action.

From Retherford, Schwartz, and Chapman in *Assessing Language Production in Children: Experimental Procedures* (p. 44) by J. Miller, 1981, Austin, TX: PRO-ED. Reprinted by permission.

**Halliday's Functions of Language.** Halliday categorized children's early uses of language in two phases: Phase I (9 to 15 months of age) and Phase II (16 to 35 months). Within the total age range, he lists seven functions of language as given below:

1. The *instrumental,* in which the *I want* function of seeking satisfaction of material needs is served by language
2. The *regulatory,* in which language serves the *Do as I tell you* function and regulates the behavior of communicative partners
3. The *interactional,* in which language serves to link *you and me* in an interaction between self and others
4. The *personal,* in which language is used for the expression of feelings and attitudes and for the personal element in interaction between communicative partners
5. The *heuristic,* in which language is used to investigate reality and to learn about things—*Tell me why.*
6. The *imaginative,* the *Let's pretend* function, in which language serves to create the child's own environment
7. The *informative,* in which language serves the function of communicating new information about something

The first six functions are exemplified in Table 5.9, which categorizes a number of Halliday's son's vocalizations at 16 to 18 months of age. Using this table, the examiner can begin to develop evaluation strategies for determining which functions a child may be using in a variety of contexts. For example, within the relatively high structure of the appraisal situation does the child produce more or fewer functions than in the mother-child context or in the peer context? Which functions are used in which context? Can unused functions within one context be elicited in that context?

Although the seven functions of language are used throughout an individual's life, Halliday identifies two principal functions during Phase II: the pragmatic and the mathetic. Apparently, older children combine the instrumental, regulatory, and interactional functions into what Halliday refers to as the general pragmatic function of speech when the symbolic system is used by the child to act on reality and becomes the language of requests. The interactional, personal, and heuristic functions combine into what Halliday terms the mathetic function, and the symbolic system is used as a means of learning about reality or reflecting it.

The reader should keep in mind that the examples shown in Table 5.9 are reflective of only one child's development and do not constitute anything approaching normative data. Other children may use Halliday's functions

## TABLE 5.9. Halliday's Functions of Language (exemplified in one child)

| Function and example | Vocalization Gloss |
|---|---|
| *Instrumental* | |
| Generalized request for object | /m/ = Give me that. |
| Request for food | *more* = I want some more. |
| | *cake* = I want some cake. |
| Request for specific objects or entertainment | *ball* = I want my ball. |
| | *Dvořak* = I want the Dvořak record on. |
| | *fish* = I want to be lifted up to where the fish picture is. |
| *Regulatory* | |
| General request for action | /ɛ/ = Do that (again). |
| Specific requests for action | *book* = Let's look at a book. |
| | *lunch* = Come for lunch. |
| Request for permission | *stick-hole* = Can I put my stick in that hole? |
| Request for assistance | /ɛ/ = Pick me up (gestures). |
| *Interactional* | |
| Greeting person | /a/ouha/ = hello |
| | *Anna* |
| Seeking person | *Anna?* = Where are you? |
| Finding person | *Anna* = There you are. |
| Initiating routines | *devil* = You say, "ooh you are the devil." |
| Expressions of shared regret | /ʔ a:/ = Let's be sad; it's broke. |
| Response to "look" | /m/ = Yes, I see. |
| Response to *where* question | /de/ = There is it. |
| *Personal* | |
| Comment on appearance of object | *star* = There's a star. |
| Comment on disappearance | *no more* = The star has gone. |
| Express feelings of: | |
| interest | /ɸ/ = That's interesting. |
| pleasure | /ayi:/ = That's nice. |
| surprise | /o/ = That's funny. |
| excitement | /ɑ/ = Look at that. |
| ritual joy | /ɛ/ = That's my ________! |
| warning | /ɥ:/ = Careful, it's sharp. |
| complaint | /ɛ:he/ = I'm fed up. |
| *Heuristic* | |
| Request for information | /ɜ$^{ad^{y}da}$/ = What's that called? |
| Acknowledgment | /m/ = I see. |
| Imitating | (imitates name) = It's a __________. |
| *Imaginative* | |
| Pretend play | (g$^{W}$ʏ\|---/ = Let's pretend to go to sleep. |
| | /ɹa::o/ = Roar; let's pretend to be a lion. |
| Jingles | *cockadoodledo* |
| *Rhymes* | (supplies final word) |

From *Learning How to Mean: Explorations in the Development of Language* (pp. 156–157) by M. Halliday, 1975, London: Edward Arnold. Reprinted by permission.

earlier or later than his son did and may not use them in the same sequence as that given.

**Dore's Primitive Speech Acts.** Dore (1975) defined a set of early "primitive" speech acts that he identified in the one-word speech of children who were just beginning to talk. These acts include labeling, repeating, answering, requesting action, requesting answers, calling, greeting, and protesting. Examples are given in Table 5.10.

The examiner may seldom or never assess children who are just beginning to speak, but it would not be unusual to assess older, nonverbal children who may produce only a few words. In such cases, Dore's framework provides a useful reference to the types of pragmatic speech acts that are common to children at very low levels of language development. In addition, the eight pragmatic categories identified in nonverbal children by Coggins and Carpenter (1978) provide clues as to pragmatic function in preverbal or nonverbal children. The categories and definitions developed by Coggins and Carpenter are shown in Table 5.11.

**Prutting-Kirchner Assessment of Pragmatic Behavior.** Prutting and Kirchner (1983) begin their description of assessment with a detailed review of school-age and adult pragmatic behaviors, organizing them within a speech act framework. According to this study, all of the behaviors should be present and used appropriately by school-age children. For the assessment of younger or developmentally delayed children, the authors refer the reader to the work of such authors as Dore (1975).

As described by Prutting and Kirchner, the utterance act is extended to include paralinguistic and nonverbal as well as verbal behaviors. The second broad behavior they describe is termed *propositional acts.* These behaviors consist of linguistic dimensions of sentence meaning and serve to orient both of the communicative partners. The third area includes the *illocutionary* and *perlocutionary* acts, which are shared behaviors regulated by the communicative partners. The illocutionary act is the speaker's intention, while the perlocutionary act is the effects of the act on the listener. Table 5.12 is an abbreviated listing of the pool of pragmatic behaviors as given in Prutting and Kirchner (1983).

Based on the pool of pragmatic behaviors, Prutting and Kirchner developed an assessment strategy, the results of which can be analyzed at two different levels: the molar and the molecular. As the authors state, assessment should be conducted for the purpose of designing therapy programs and should be no more detailed than is necessary for designing the program.

The protocol is organized around four areas: the utterance act, the propositional act, the illocutionary act, and the perlocutionary act. Observation of the child's pragmatic behaviors can indicate where the problem

## TABLE 5.10. Dore's Primitive Speech Acts

| Speech act | Definition | Example |
|---|---|---|
| *Labeling* | Uses word while attending to object or event. Does not address adult or wait for a response. | C touches a doll's eyes and says *eyes.* |
| *Repeating* | Repeats part or all of prior adult utterance. Does not wait for a response. | C overhears Mother's utterance of *doctor* and says *doctor.* |
| *Answering* | Answers adult's question. Addresses adult. | Mother points to a picture of a dog and asks *What's that?* C answers *bow-wow.* |
| *Requesting action* | Word or vocalization often accompanied by gesture signaling demand. Addresses adult and awaits response. | C, unable to push a peg through hole, utters *uh uh uh* while looking at Mother. |
| *Requesting* | Asks question with a word, sometimes accompanying gesture. Addresses adult and awaits response. | C picks up book, looks at Mother, and says *book?* with rising terminal contour. Mother answers *Right, it's a book.* |
| *Calling* | Calls adult's name loudly and awaits response. | C shouts *mama* to his mother across the room. |
| *Greeting* | Greets adult or object upon its appearance. | C says *hi* when teacher enters room. |
| *Protesting* | Resists adult's action with word or cry. Addresses adult. | C, when his mother attempts to put on his shoe, utters an extended scream of varying contours while resisting her. |
| *Practicing* | Use of word or prosodic pattern in absence of any specific object or event. Does not address adult. Does not await response. | C utters *Daddy* when he is not present. |

From "Holophrases, Speech Acts, and Language Universals" by J. Dore, 1975, *Journal of Child Language, 2,* pp. 21–40. Reprinted by permission.

**TABLE 5.11. Pragmatic Behaviors in Nonverbal Children**

| Category | Definition |
|---|---|
| *Requesting* | Solicitation of a service from a listener: |
| *Object* requests | Gestures or utterances that direct the listener to provide some object for the child |
| *Action* requests | Gestures or utterances that direct the listener to act upon some object in order to make it move. The action, rather than the object, is the focus of the child's interest. |
| *Information* requests | Gestures or utterances that direct the listener to provide information about an object, action, or location |
| *Greeting* | Gestures or utterances subsequent to a person's entrance that express recognition |
| *Transferring* | Gestures intended to place an object in another person's possession |
| *Showing off* | Gestures or utterances that appear to be used to attract attention |
| *Acknowledging* | Gestures or utterances that provide notice that the listener's previous utterances were received |
| *Answering* | Gestures or utterances from the child in response to a request for information from the listener |

lies. It may be at any one level or across levels, and difficulties at one level may lead to difficulties at another. For example, if the child has a problem with propositional acts (linguistic dimensions of sentence meaning), it is more likely that problems will be noted in conversational interaction than if he or she has a problem at the utterance level.

The examiner should always be aware that a pragmatic deficit can occur in combination with linguistic or cognitive deficits or may occur in isolation from other deficits. There is no evidence as to the incidence of pragmatic deficits either in isolation or in combination with other problems, and according to Prutting and Kirchner, there is no good evidence whether a pragmatic deficit would or should qualify as a legitimate problem needing therapeutic attention. At this time individual clinicians must decide for themselves whether the time needed to assess pragmatic behaviors is worth the results.

**TABLE 5.12. Pool of Pragmatic Behaviors**

| Taxonomy | Modality | Description and Coding |
|---|---|---|
| UTTERANCE ACT | Verbal/paralinguistic | the trappings by which the act is accomplished |
| 1. Intelligibility | | the extent to which the message is understood |
| 1. Intelligibility | | |
| 4. Prosody | | the intonation and stress patterns of the message |
| 6. Physical contacts | Nonverbal | the distance which speaker and listener sit or stand from one another |
| PROPOSITIONAL ACT | Verbal | linguistic dimension of the meaning of the sentence |
| 1. Lexical selection/use | | |
| A. specificity/accuracy | | lexical items of best fit considering the context |
| 2. Specifying relationships between words | | |
| A. Word order | | grammatical word order for conveying message |
| ILLOCUTIONARY AND PERLOCUTIONARY ACTS | Verbal | intentions of the speaker and effects on the listener |
| 1. Speech act pair analysis | | the ability to take both speaker and listener role appropriate to the context |
| B. Turntaking | | smooth interchanges between speaker and listener |

From "Applied Pragmatics" by C. Prutting and D. Kirchner, 1983, *Pragmatic Assessment and Intervention Issues in Language,* edited by T. Gallagher and C. Prutting, San Diego: College-Hill Press. Reprinted by permission.

## SUMMARY

This chapter has dealt with the informal assessment of oral language production—namely, the examination of the oral speech mechanism; assessment or articulatory proficiency; and the assessment of syntax, semantics, and pragmatics in oral production. As indicated previously, the assessment strategies reviewed are generally not normative and, in some instances, are based on only minimal developmental data. In no way does informal assessment take the place of standardized evaluation, except with children too young or too severely handicapped to be assessed with standardized instruments. For this reason, some of the well-standardized measures have been reviewed.

The procedure that we continue to suggest is: (a) Administer well-standardized, appropriate measures of language ability to determine whether a problem actually exists, (b) assess children in areas of deficit using strategies such as those discussed above to determine and design a therapeutic program, and (c) design the therapeutic program using the assessment information gained to determine a starting place for therapy and to measure progress. There should be no real quarrel between the advocates of standardized testing and advocates of informal assessment. There is a place for both, and both are equally valuable.

## REFERENCES

Angler, L., Hannah, E. P., & Longhurst, T. M. (1973). Linguistic analysis of speech samples: A practical guide for clinicians. *Journal of Speech and Hearing Disorders, 38,* 192–204.

Aungst, L., & Frick, J. (1964). Auditory discrimination ability and consistency of articulation of /r/. *Journal of Speech and Hearing Disorders, 29,* 76–85.

Bangs, T. E. (1977). *Vocabulary Comprehension Scale.* Dallas: Developmental Learning Materials.

Bangs, T., & Dodson, D. (1979). *Birth to Three Developmental Scale.* Dallas: Developmental Learning Materials.

Bellugi-Klima, U. (1971). Some language comprehension tests. In C. Lavatelli (Ed.), *Language training in early childhood education* (pp. 157–170). Urbana, IL: University of Illinois Press.

Bloom, L. (1970). *Language development: Form and function in emerging grammars.* Cambridge, MA: MIT Press.

Bloom, L. (1973). *One word at a time.* The Hague: Mouton.

Bloom, L., & Lahey, M. (1978). *Language development and language disorders.* New York: John Wiley.

Brown, R. (1970). The first sentences of child and chimpanzee. In R. Brown (Ed.), *Psycholinguistics.* New York: Free Press.

Brown, R. (1973). *A first language: The early stages.* Cambridge, MA: Harvard University Press.

Bryant, B., & Bryant, D. (1983). *Test of Articulation Performance–Diagnostic.* Austin, TX: PRO-ED.

Bryen, D. N. (1974). Special education and the linguistically different child. *Exceptional Children, 40,* 589–599.

Carrow, E. (1973). *Test for Auditory Comprehension of Language.* New York: Teaching Resources.

Carrow, E. (1974). *Carrow Elicited Language Inventory.* New York: Teaching Resources.

Clark, J. B., & Madison, C. L. (1981). *Clark-Madison Test of Oral Language.* Tigard, OR: C.C. Publications.

Coggins, T., & Carpenter, R. (1978). Categories for coding pre-speech intentional communication. Unpublished manuscript, University of Washington, Seattle.

Compton, A. (1970). Generative studies of children's phonological disorders. *Journal of Speech and Hearing Disorders, 35,* 315–339.

de Villiers, J., & de Villiers, P. (1973). A cross-sectional study of the acquisition of grammatical morphemes in child speech. *Journal of Psycholinguistic Research, 2,* 267–268.

Dore, J. (1975). Holophrases, speech acts, and language universals. *Journal of Child Language, 2,* 21–40.

Dunn, L. (1981). *Peabody Picture Vocabulary Test.* Circle Pines, MN: American Guidance Service.

Englemann, S. (1967). *Basic Concept Inventory.* Chicago: Follett.

Fewell, R., & Langley, M. (1984). *Developmental Activities Screening Inventory.* Austin, TX: PRO-ED.

Fisher, H., & Logemann, J. (1971). *Fisher-Logemann Test of Articulation Competence.* Boston: Houghton Mifflin.

Foster, C. R., Giddan, J. J., & Stark, J. (1972). *Assessment of Children's Language Comprehension.* Palo Alto, CA: Consulting Psychologists Press.

Frankenburg, W., Dodds, J., Fandal, A., Kazuk, E., & Cohrs, M. (1975). *Denver Developmental Screening Test.* Denver: LADOCA.

Gallagher, T. (1983). Pre-assessment: A procedure for accommodating language use variability. In T. Gallagher & C. Prutting (Eds.), *Pragmatic assessment and intervention issues in language* (pp. 1–29). San Diego: College-Hill Press.

Goldman, R., & Fristoe, M. (1969). *Goldman-Fristoe Test of Articulation.* Circle Pines, MN: American Guidance Service.

Greenfield, P., & Smith, J. (1976). *The structure of communication in early language development.* New York: Academic Press.

Halliday, M. (1975). *Learning how to mean: Explorations in the development of language.* London: Edward Arnold.

Hammill, D. D., Brown, V. L., Larsen, S. C., & Wiederholt, J. L. (1987). *Test of Adolescent Language.* Austin, TX: PRO-ED.

Hammill, D. D., & Newcomer, P. L. (1982). *Test of Language Development–Primary.* Austin, TX: PRO-ED.

Hresko, W. P., Reid, D. K., & Hammill, D. D. (1981). *The Test of Early Language Development.* Austin, TX: PRO-ED.

Ingram, D. (1976). *Phonological disability in children.* London: Edward Arnold.

Ireton, H., & Thwing, E. (1972). *Minnesota Child Development Inventory.* Minneapolis, MN: Behavior Science Systems.

Jakobson, R., Fant, G., & Halle, M. (1963). *Preliminaries to speech analysis.* Cambridge, MA: MIT Press.

Kirk, S., McCarthy, M., & Kirk, W. (1968). *Illinois Test of Psycholinguistic Abilities.* Urbana, IL: University of Illinois Press.

Lee, L. (1969). *Northwestern Syntax Screening Test.* Evanston, IL: Northwestern University Press.

Lee, L. (1974). *Developmental Sentence Analysis.* Evanston, IL: Northwestern University Press.

Loban, W. (1976). *Language development.* Urbana, IL: National Council of Teachers of English.

McCarthy, D. (1930). *The language development of the preschool child* (Institute of Child Welfare Monographs Series No. 4). Minneapolis, MN: University of Minnesota.

McDonald, E. (1964). *A Deep Test of Articulation.* Tucson, AZ: Communication Skill Builders.

McReynolds, L., & Huston, K. (1971). A distinctive feature analysis of children's misarticulations. *Journal of Speech and Hearing Disorders, 36,* 155–166.

Mecham, M. (1958). *Verbal Language Development Scale.* Circle Pines, MN: American Guidance Service.

Mecham, M., Jex, J., & Jones, J. (1973). *Utah Test of Language Development.* Austin, TX: PRO-ED.

Miller, J. (1981). *Assessing language production in children: Experimental procedures.* Austin, TX: PRO-ED.

Miller, J., & Yoder, D. (1984). *Miller-Yoder Test of Grammatical Comprehension.* Austin, TX: PRO-ED.

Newcomer, P. L., & Hammill, D. D. (1982). *Test of Language Development#Intermediate.* Austin, TX: PRO-ED.

Pollack, E., & Rees, N. (1972). Disorders of articulation: Some clinical applications of distinctive feature theory. *Journal of Speech and Hearing Disorders, 37,* 451–461.

Powers, M. (1957). Functional disorders of articulation: Symptomatology and etiology. In L. Travis (Ed.), *Handbook of speech pathology* (pp. 98–131). New York: Appleton-Century-Crofts.

Prutting, C., & Kirchner, D. (1983). Applied pragmatics. In T. Gallagher & C. Prutting (Eds.), *Pragmatic assessment and intervention issues in language* (pp. 29–65). San Diego: College-Hill Press.

Sanders, L. (1972). *Procedural guides for evaluation of speech and language disorders in children.* Danville, IL: Interstate.

Schane, S. (1973). *Generative phonology.* Englewood Cliffs, NJ: Prentice-Hall.

Schlesinger, I. (1971). Production of utterances and language acquisition. In D. Slobin (Ed.), *The onotogenesis of grammar* (pp. 63–101). New York: Academic Press.

Semel, E., & Wiig, E. (1980). *Clinical Evaluation of Language Functions–Diagnostic Battery.* San Antonio, TX: Psychological Corporation.

Shriberg, L., & Kwiatkowski, J. (1980). *Natural process analysis: A procedure for phonological analysis of continuous speech samples.* New York: John Wiley.

Slobin, D. (1967). *A field manual for cross-cultural study of the acquisition of communicative competence.* Berkeley, CA: University of California Press.

Templin, M. (1957). *Certain language skills in children* (Institute of Child Welfare Monograph Series No. 26). Minneapolis, MN: University of Minnesota Press.

Templin, M., & Darley, F. (1969). *The Templin-Darley Tests of Articulation* (2nd ed.). Iowa City, IA: Bureau of Educational Research and Service, University of Iowa.

Toronto, A. S. (1973). *Screening Test of Spanish Grammar.* Evanston, IL: Northwestern University Press.

Van Riper, C. (1963). *Speech correction: Principles and methods.* Englewood Cliffs, NJ: Prentice-Hall.

Wepman, J. (1958). *Auditory Discrimination Test.* Los Angeles: Western Psychological Service.